The Adventures of Coco in Dinosaur Valley

Story by
Christine Ann Gowey

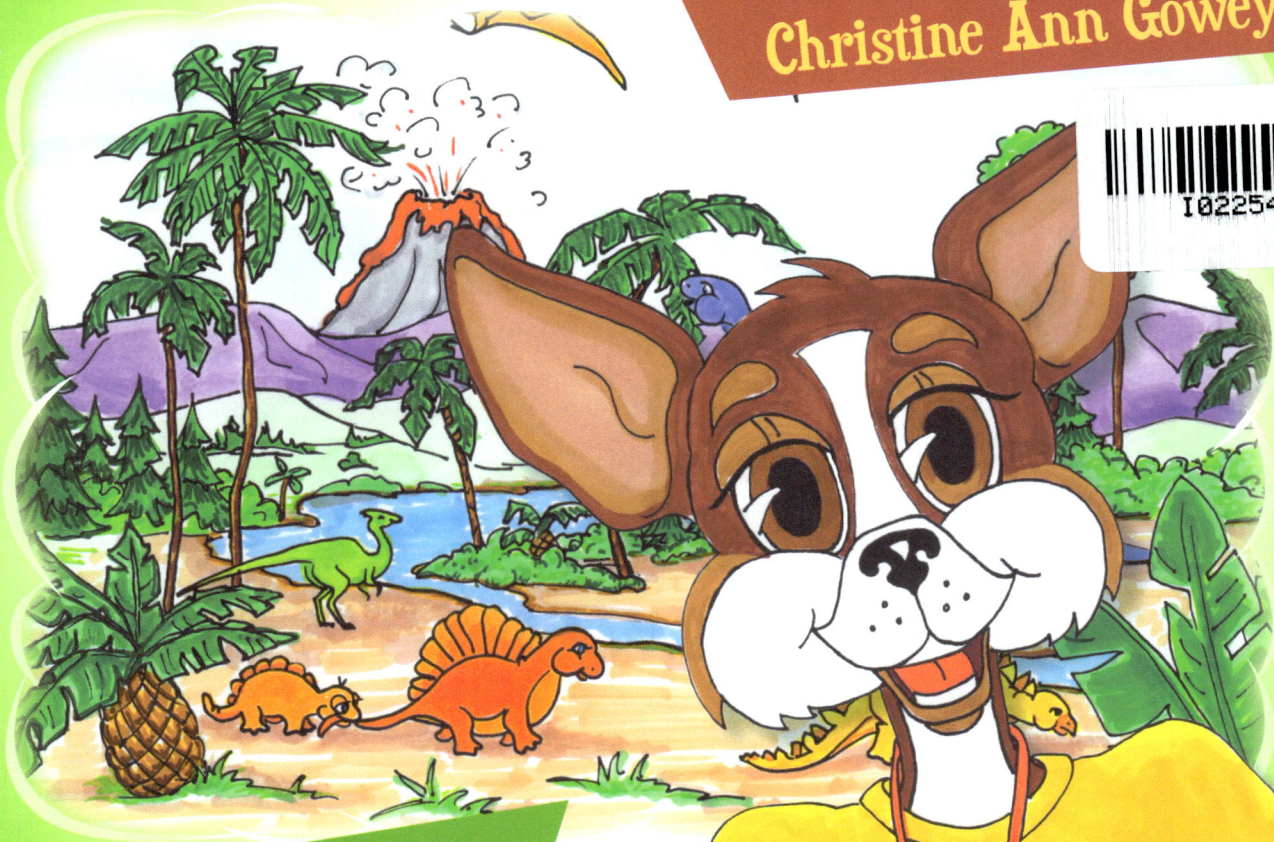

Illustrations by
Andi Kleinman

with a Special Message from
Dr. Brandie Gowey, NMD

Introducing, Coco!

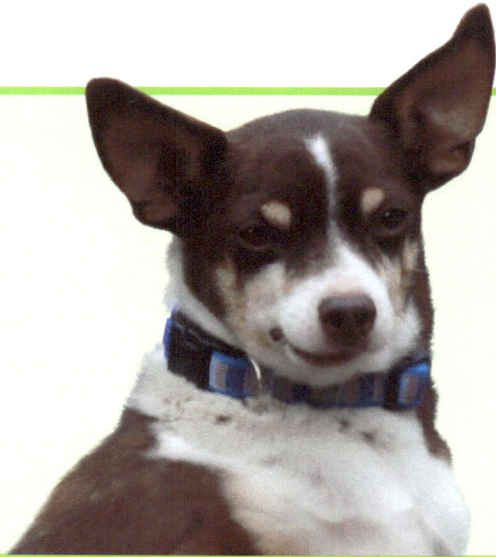

Meet the amazing Coco, the feisty little guy with a **BIG HEART** whose antics inspired the author to write about adventures Coco dreams he could have!

The Adventures of Coco in Dinosaur Valley

© 2017 by Christine Gowey, Andi Kleinman, Brandie Gowey

Published by
DR. DNA Press
Flagstaff, AZ

ISBN: 978-0-9861850-6-9

Nation of Publication: United States of America

Proceeds from the sale of this book benefit medical research at DR. DNA Clinic.
Learn more at *goweyresearchgroup.com*.

Edited by
Charlotte Fox
Dr. Brandie Gowey, NMD

Cover & Book Design by
Andi Kleinman

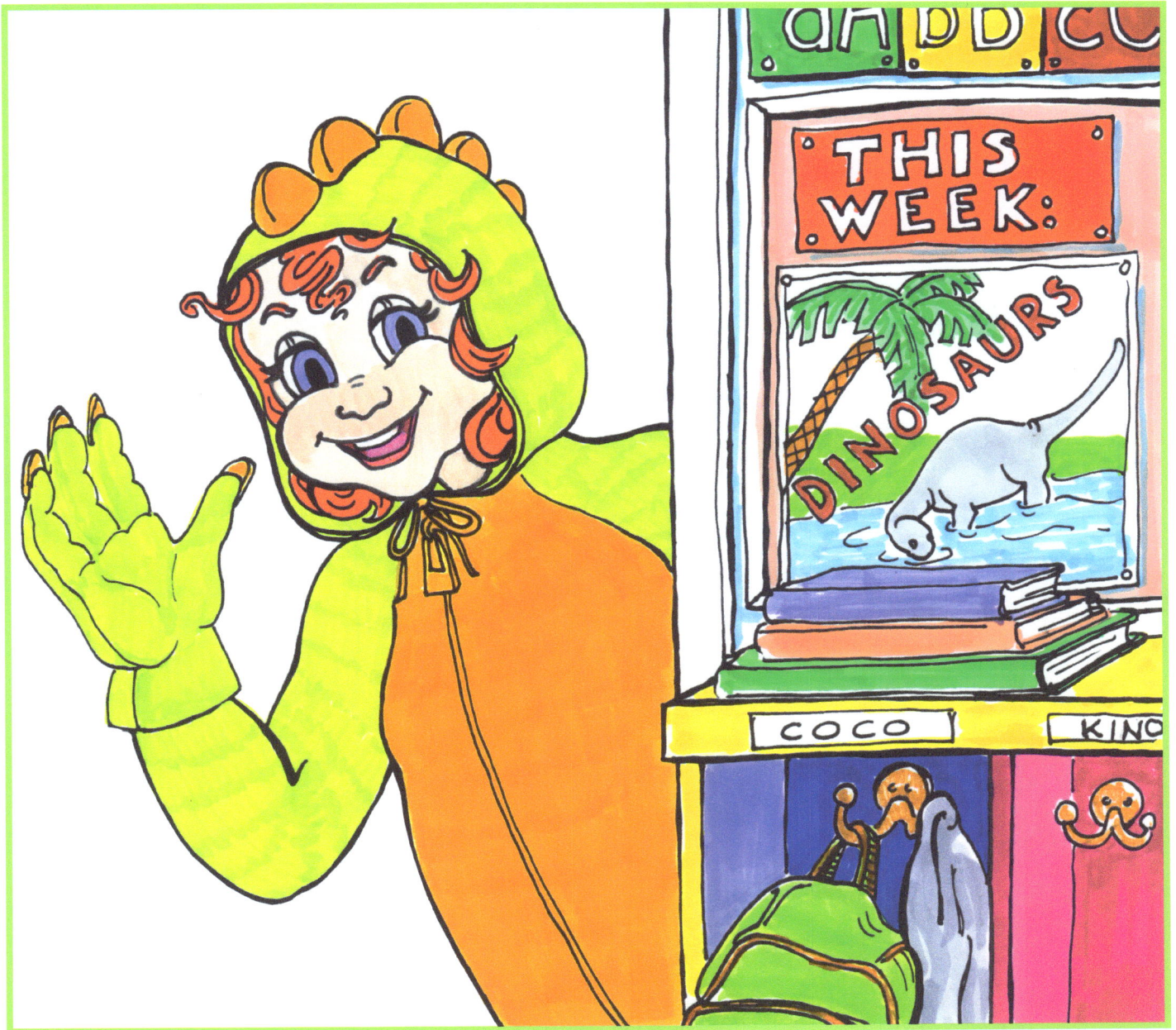

Mrs. Jabbers was sillier than usual this morning. She peeked around the corner of her classroom door wearing a dinosaur costume! Coco became very excited for today's lesson on dinosaurs!

1

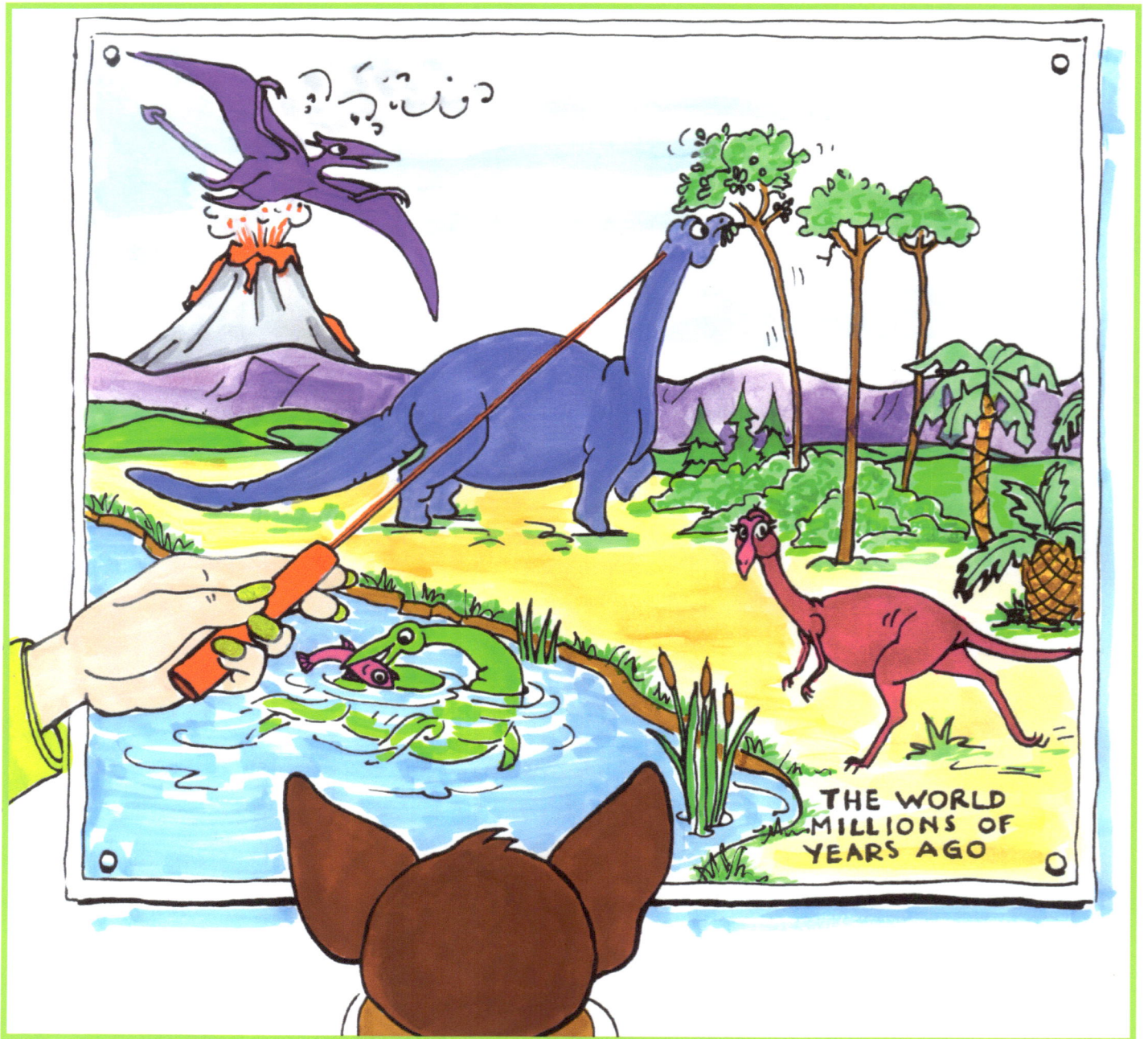

Mrs. Jabbers began to tell the class about the dinosaurs
that roamed the earth millions of years ago.

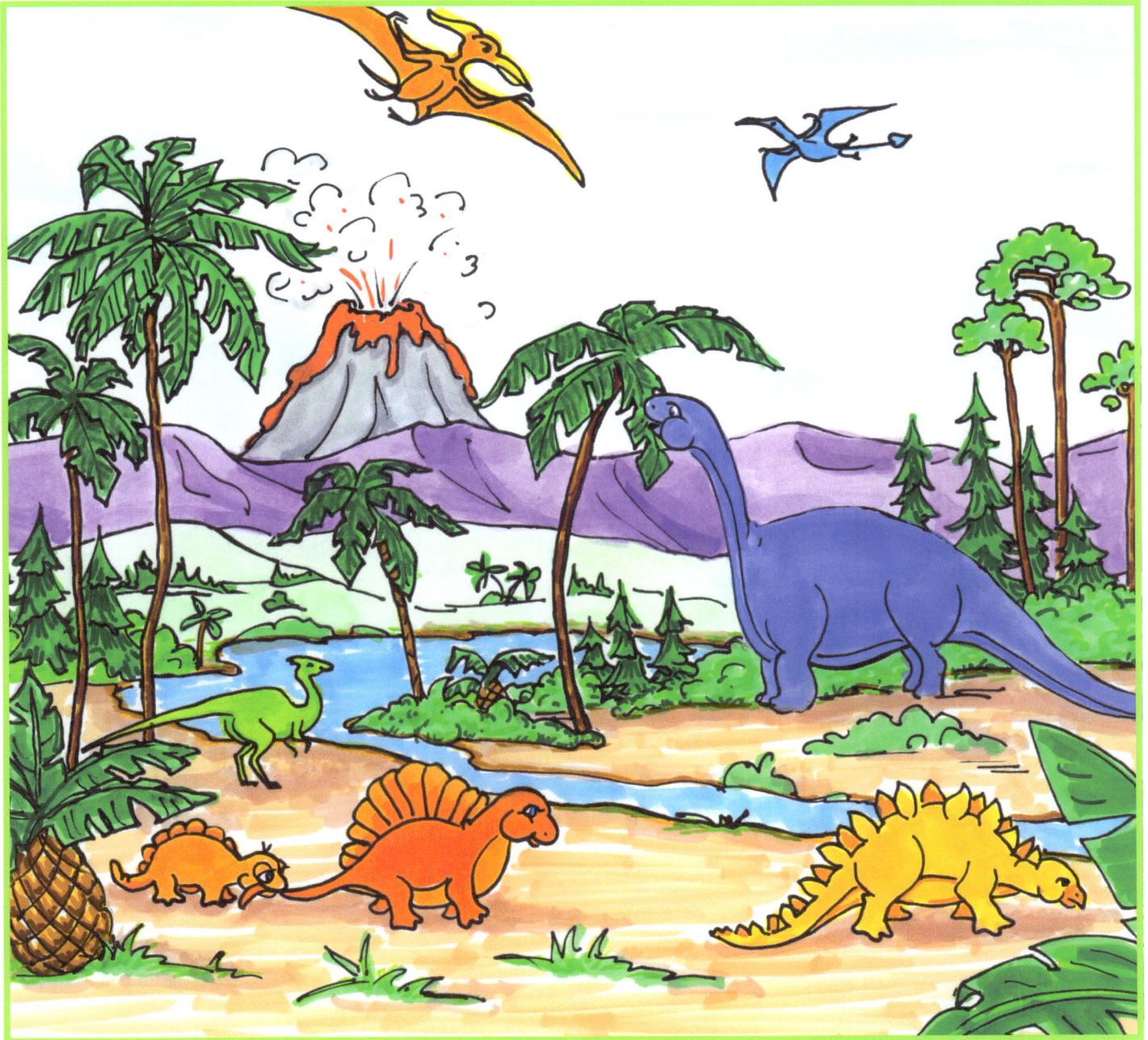

"There were dinosaurs of every size, shape, and skill.
Many of them liked to swim in water and then sun themselves…"

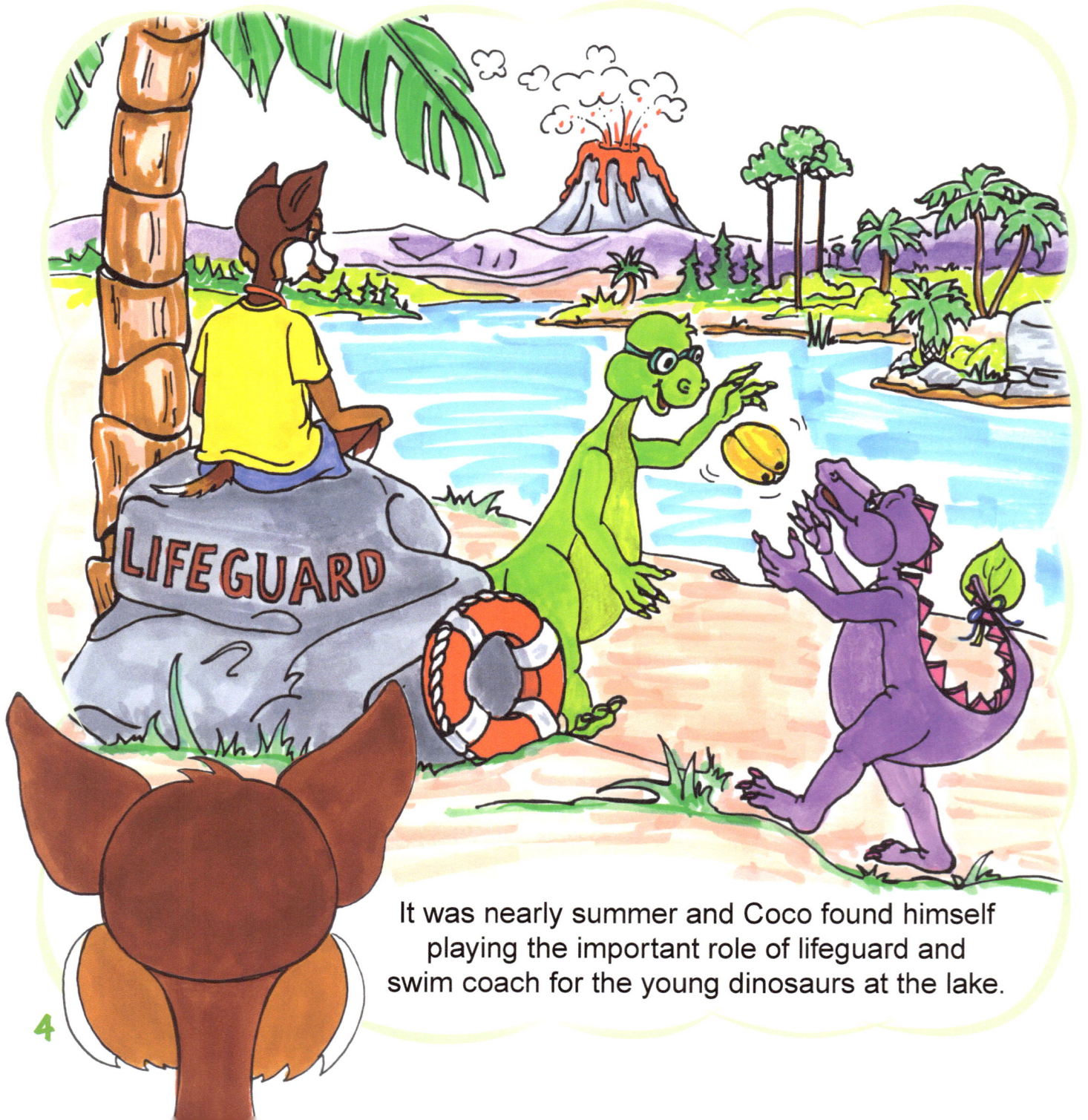

It was nearly summer and Coco found himself playing the important role of lifeguard and swim coach for the young dinosaurs at the lake.

The first thing Coco taught his students was to listen and always be safe. "Okay, class, before we hit the water, we need to go over a few rules. Who can tell me what we must always remember?"

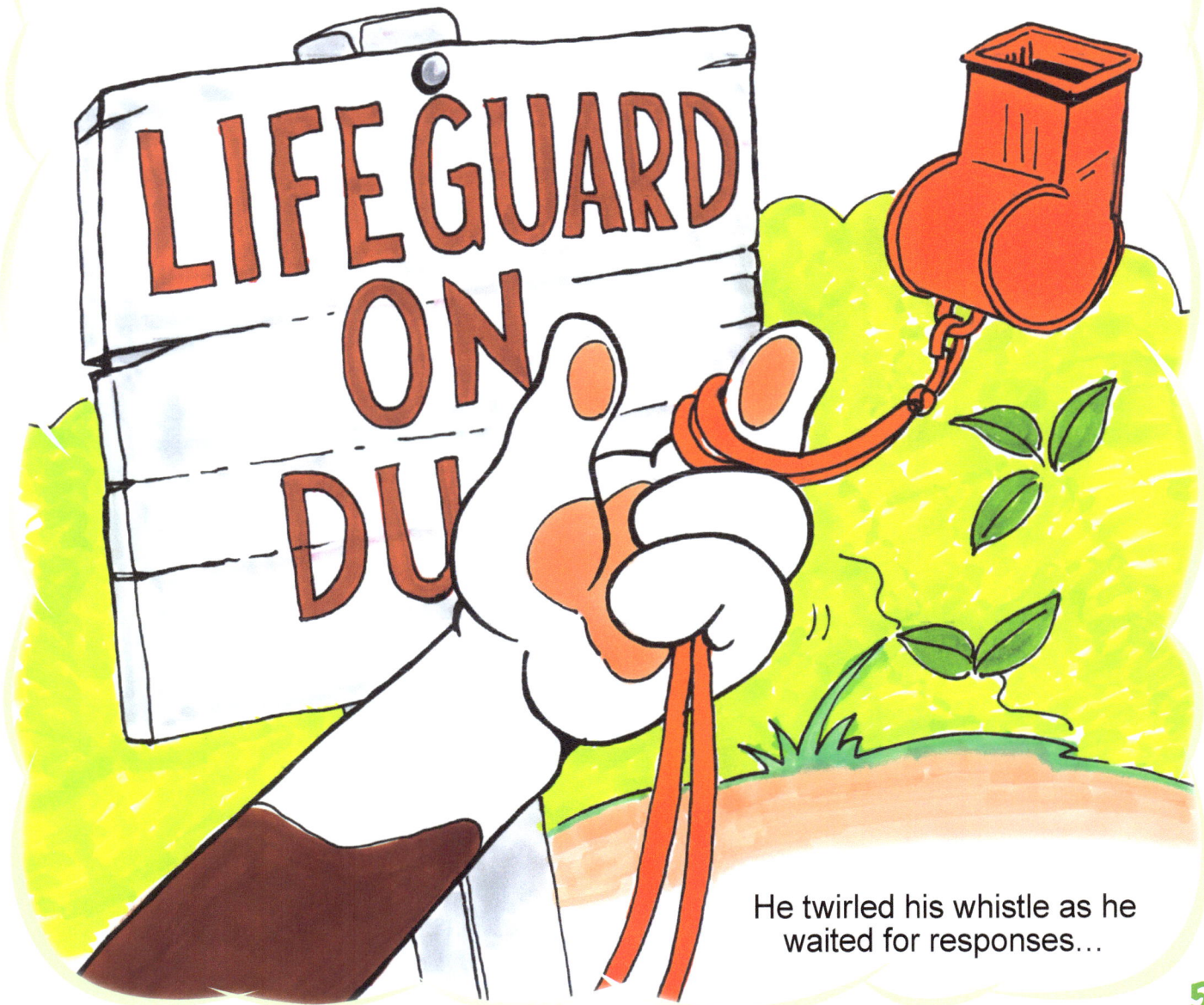

He twirled his whistle as he waited for responses…

Soon Thunder, the smallest of the group, wagged his tail and said, "Always swim with a buddy."

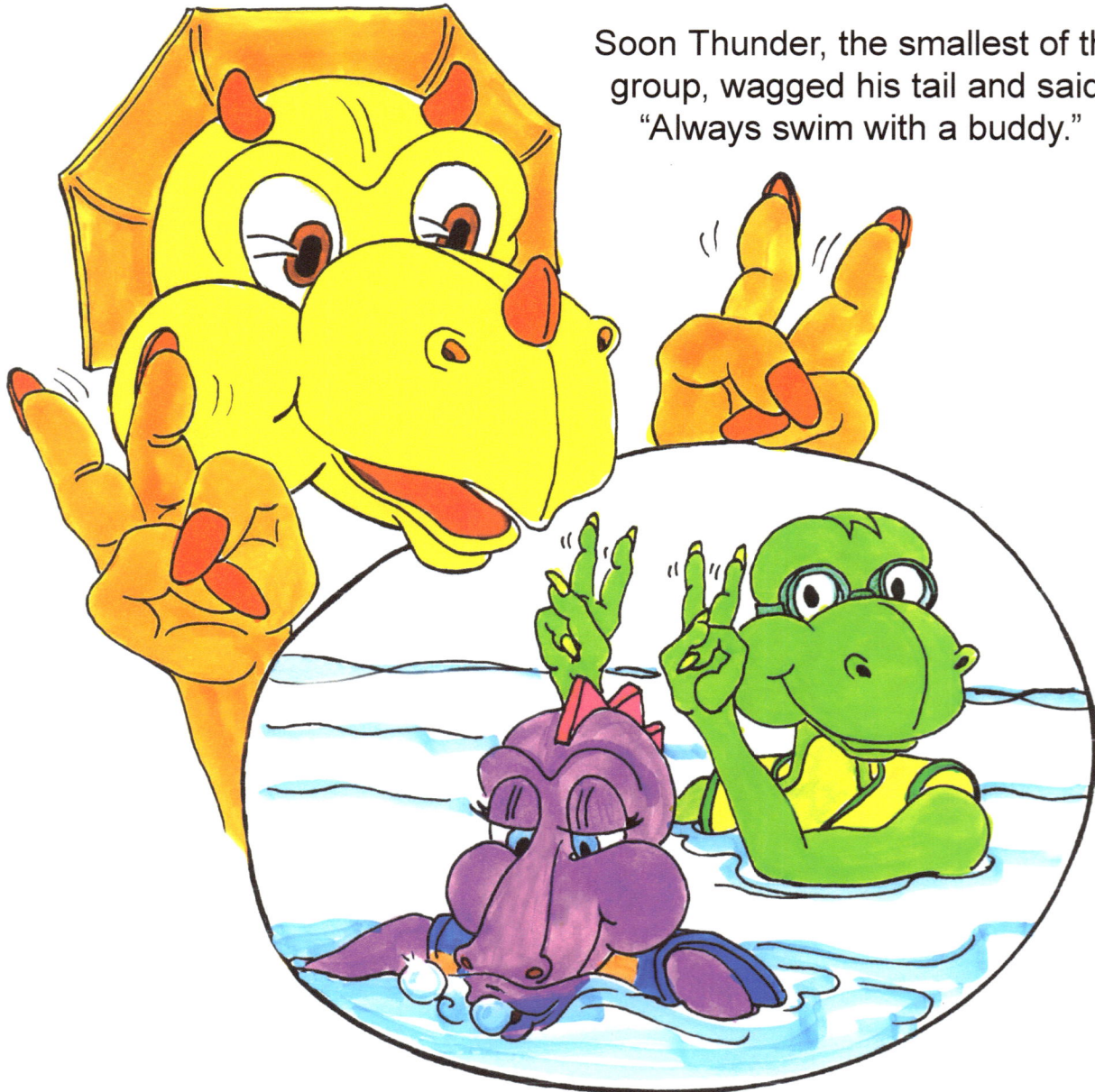

"Excellent, Thunder! Can anyone think of any more safety rules?"

Fan Tail Fay said,
"Always walk, never run—
especially on slick rock!"

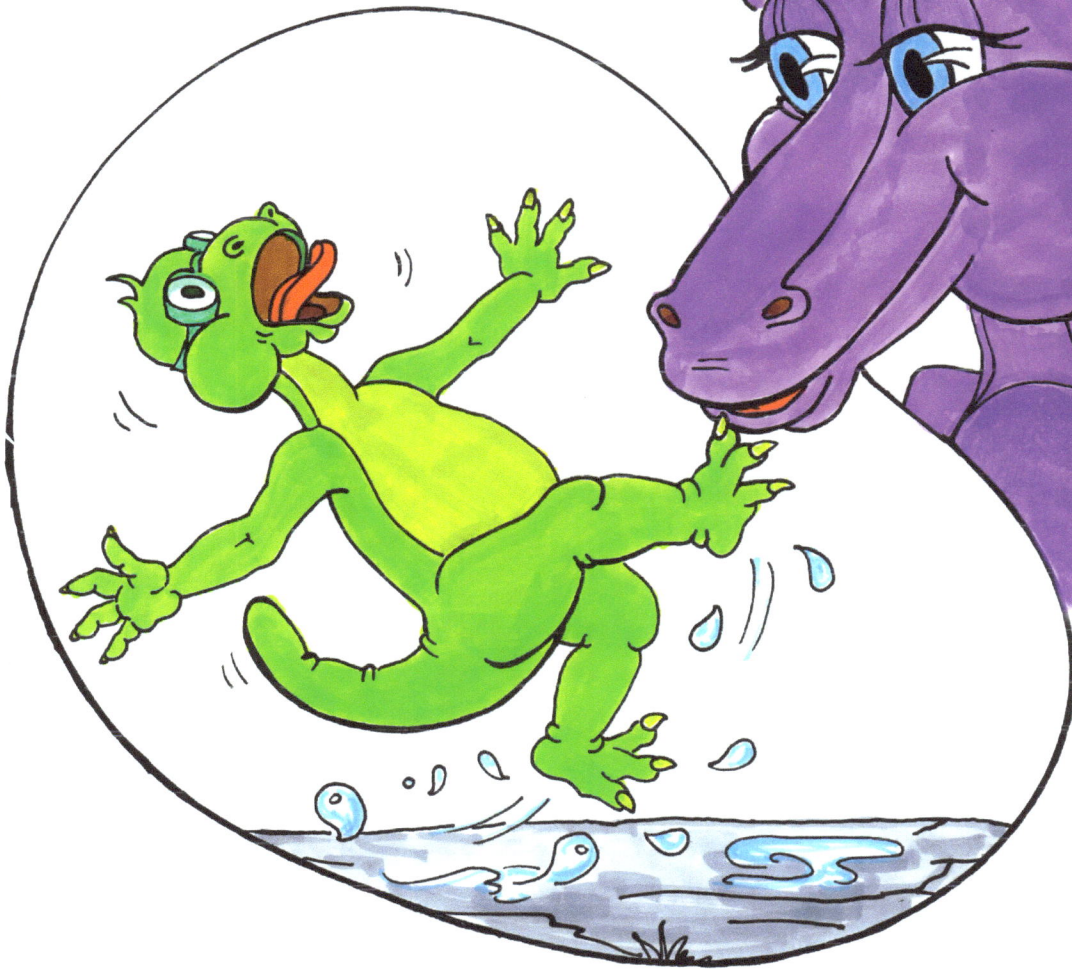

"Good one, Fan Tail Fay! Can anyone think of another?"

Bammer chimed in with "Always ask grown-ups for help if another dinosaur is in trouble in the water."

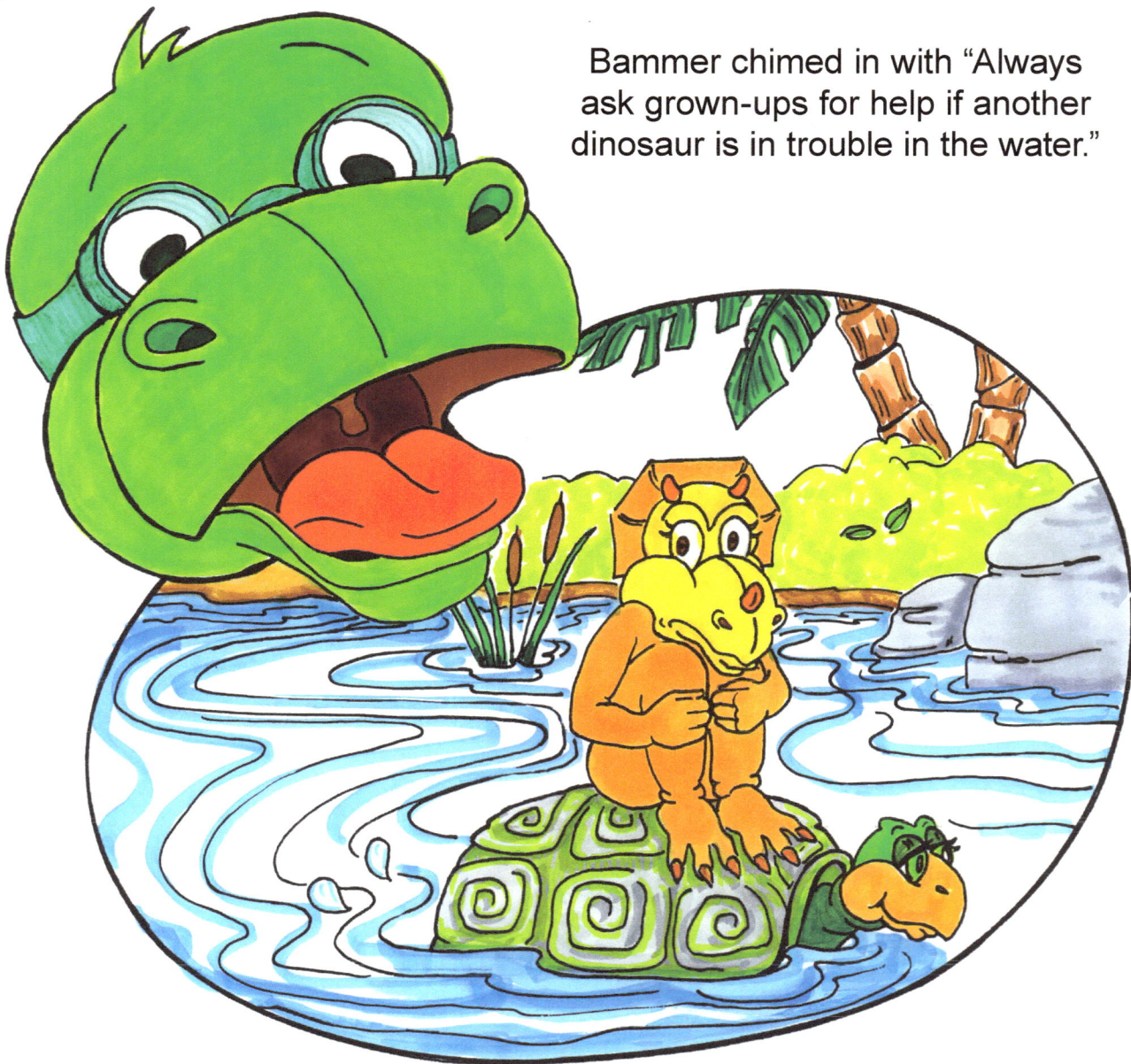

Coco smiled and said, "Excellent, Bammer!"

He then continued,
"If you have
sunscreen on today,
wave your tails!"

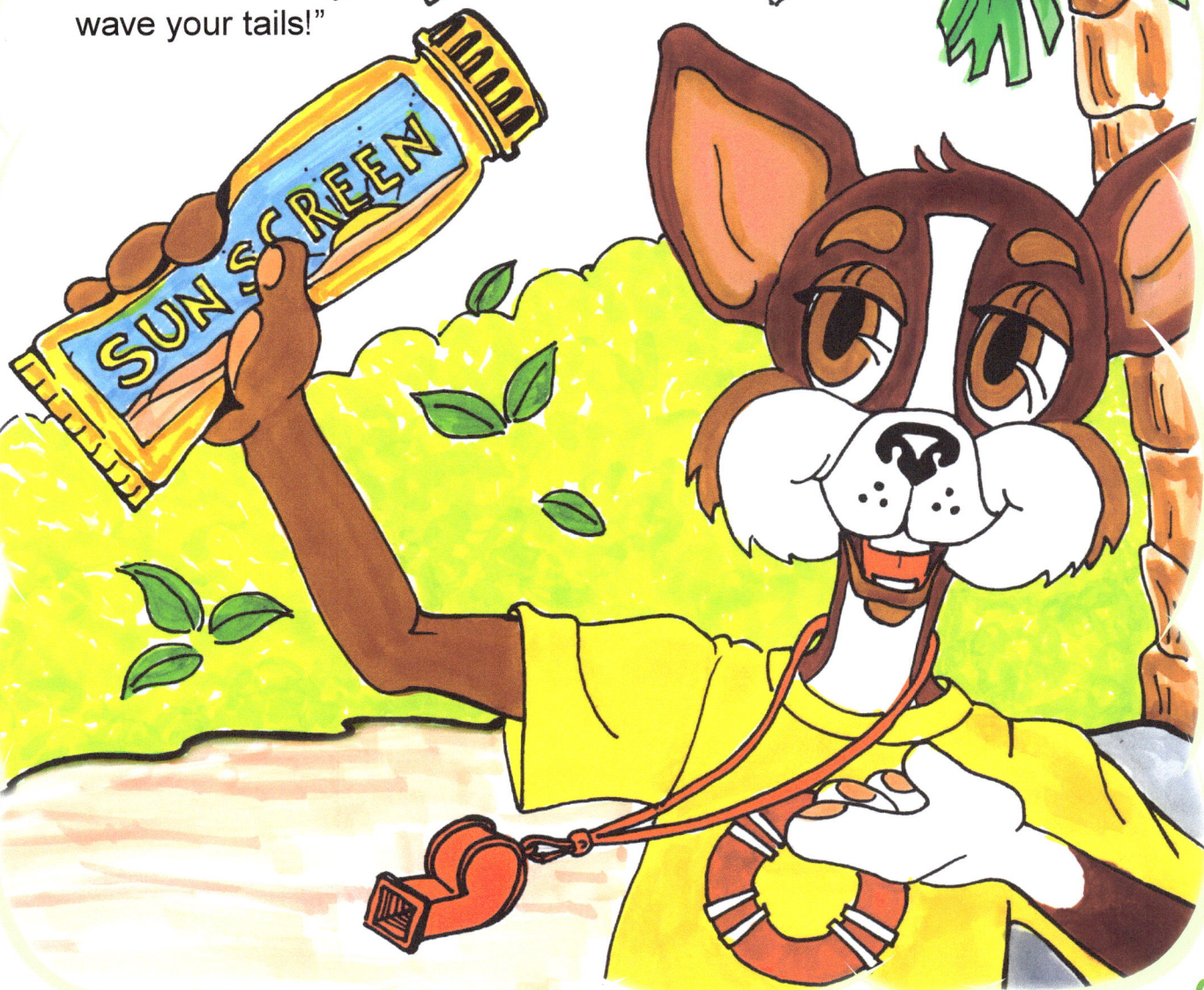

Every tail waved.

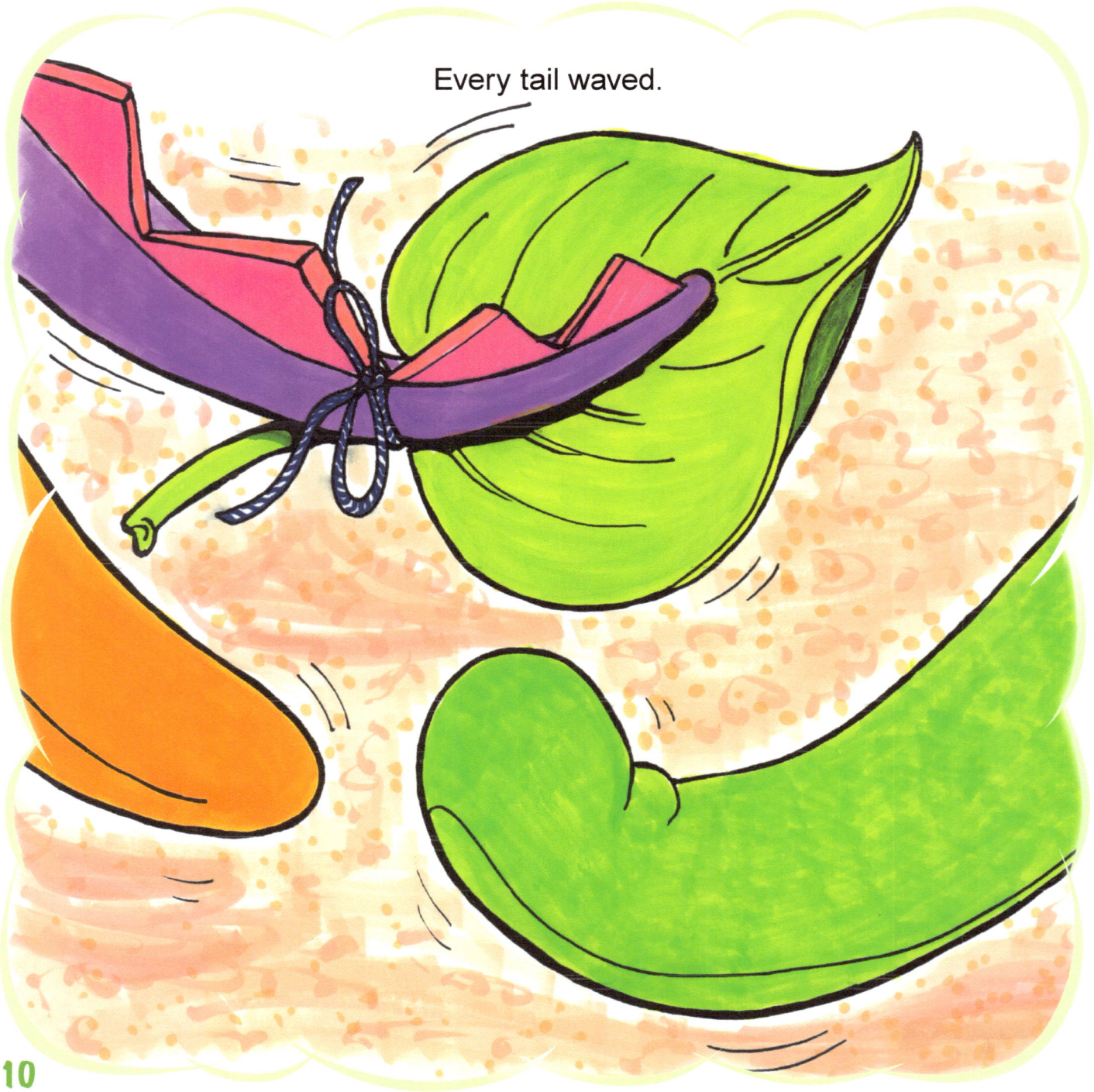

"Good! Now let's get on our life jackets," Coco said.

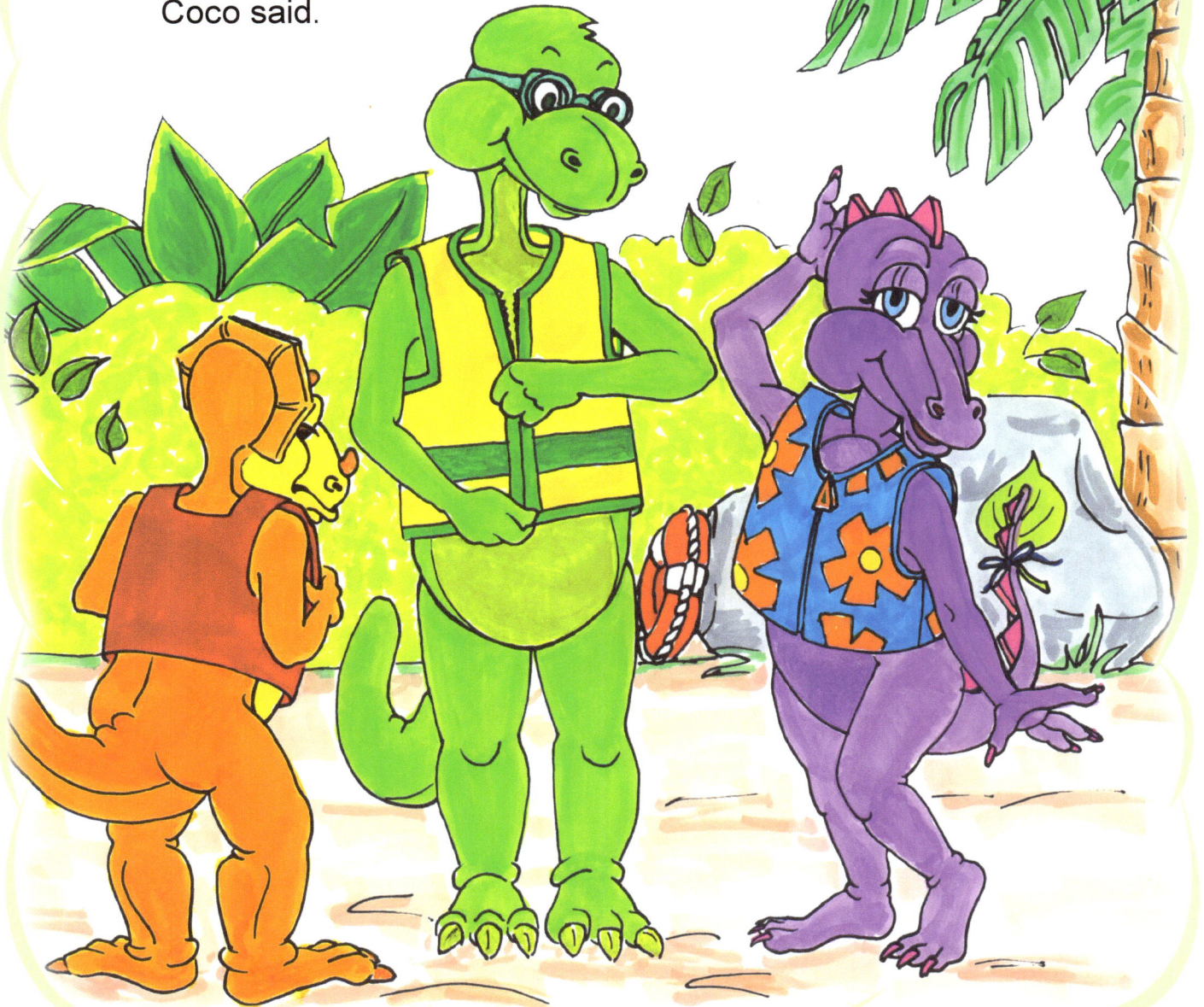

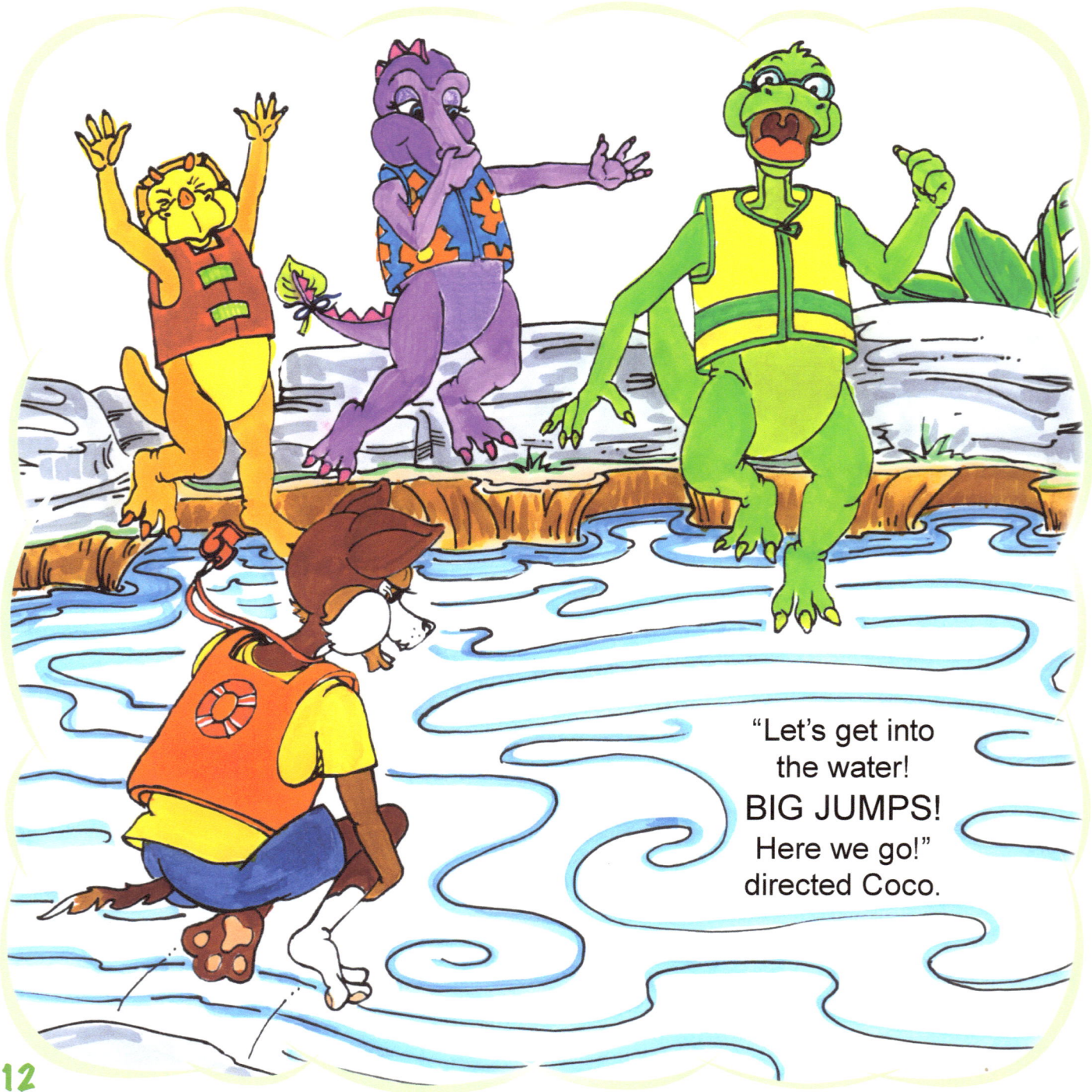

"Let's get into
the water!
BIG JUMPS!
Here we go!"
directed Coco.

Everybody jumped! The water went everywhere. (As a matter of fact, all the water splashed out of the lake…then it splashed back in!) Laughter was heard throughout the canyon.

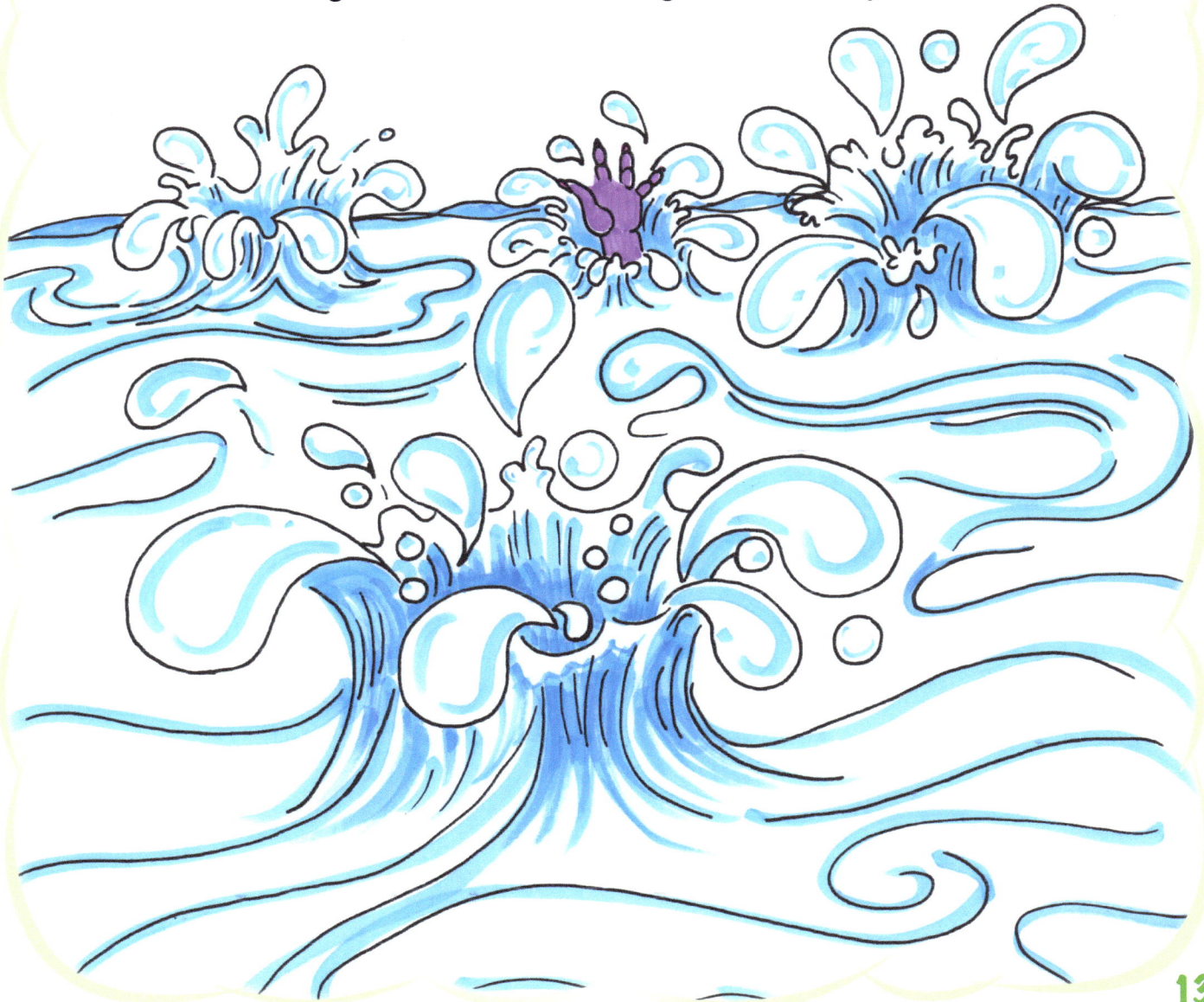

Coco showed his students
how to bob and blow bubbles...

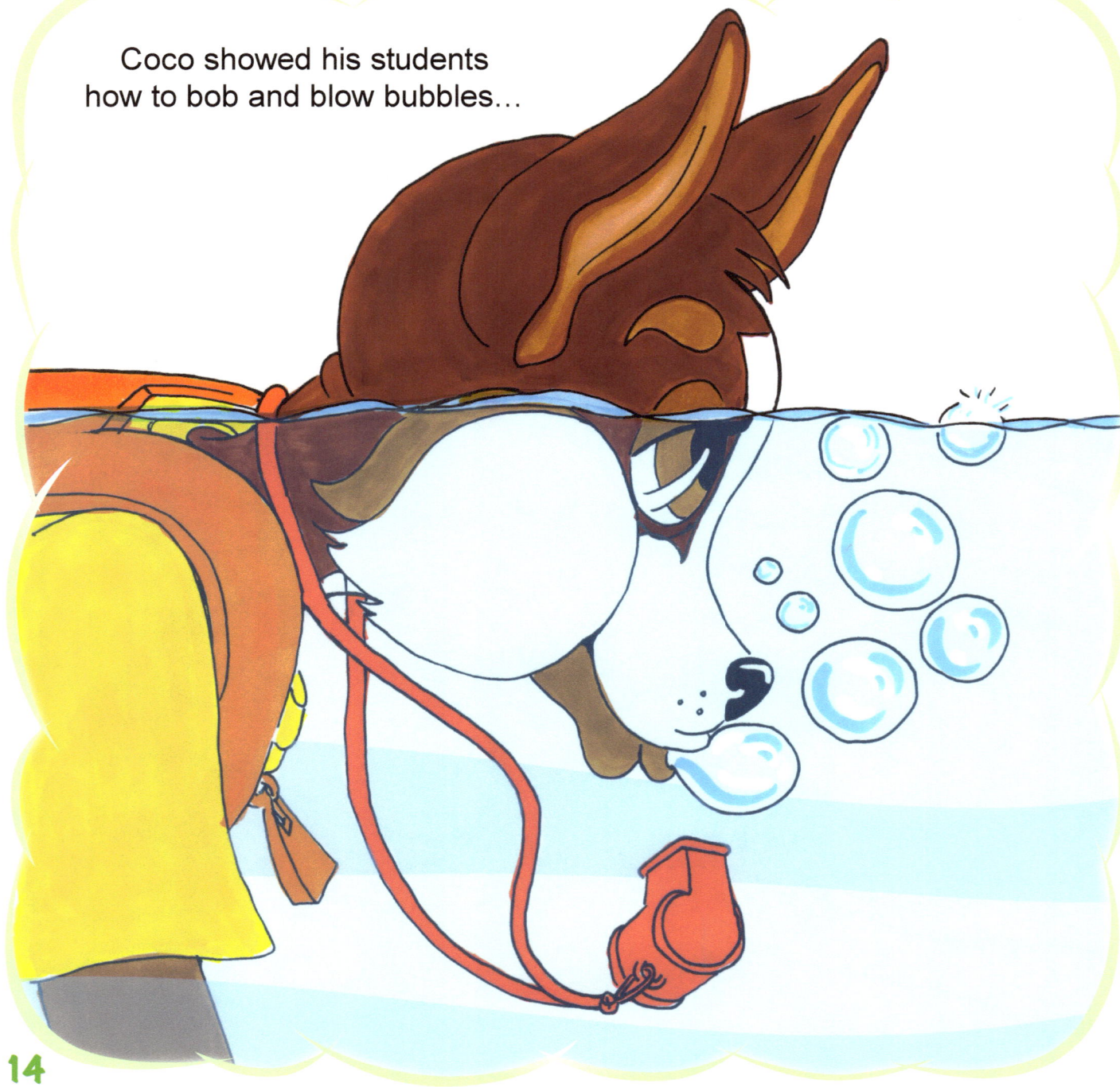

…how to breathe on their fronts…

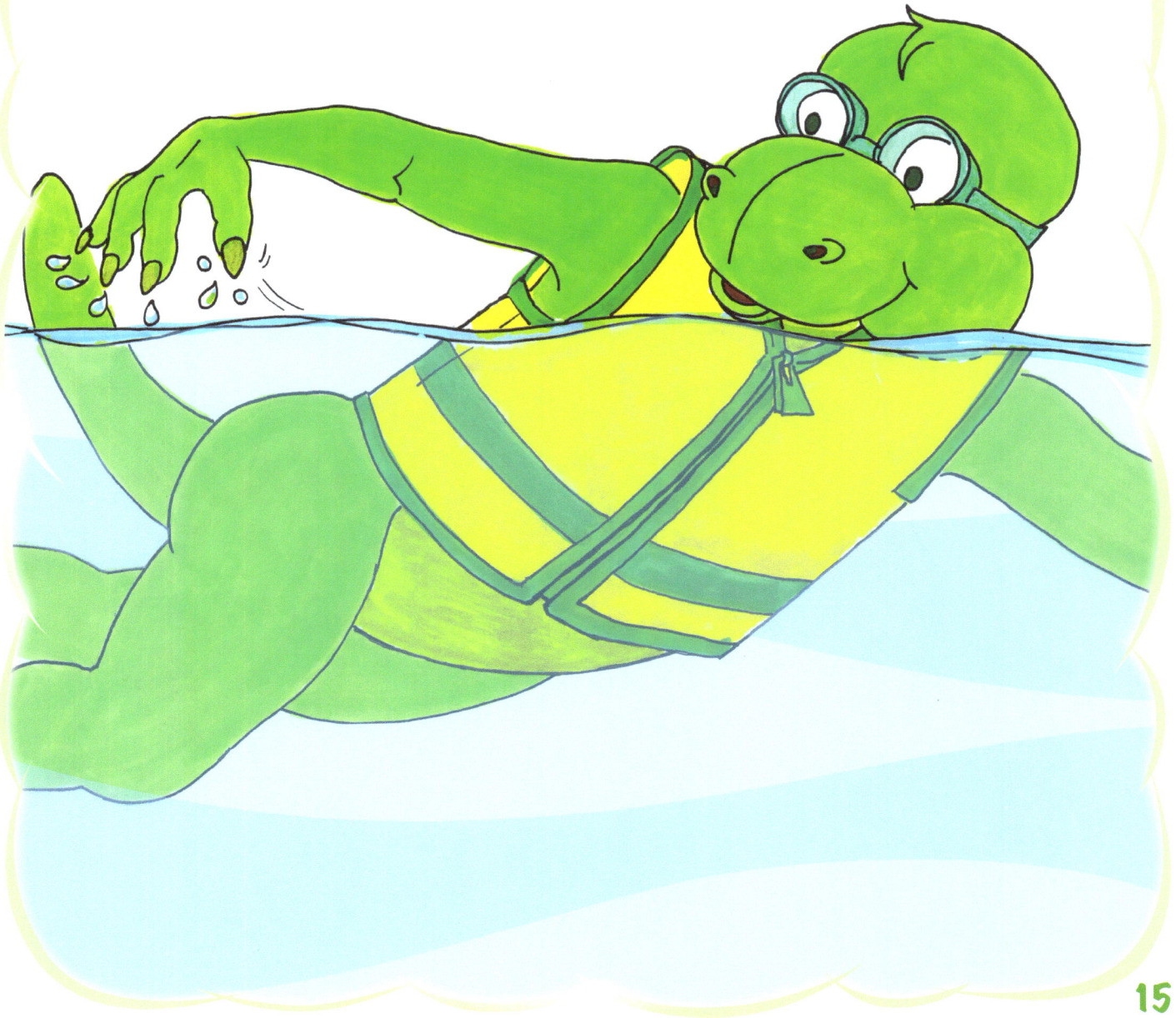

…and how to float on their backs.

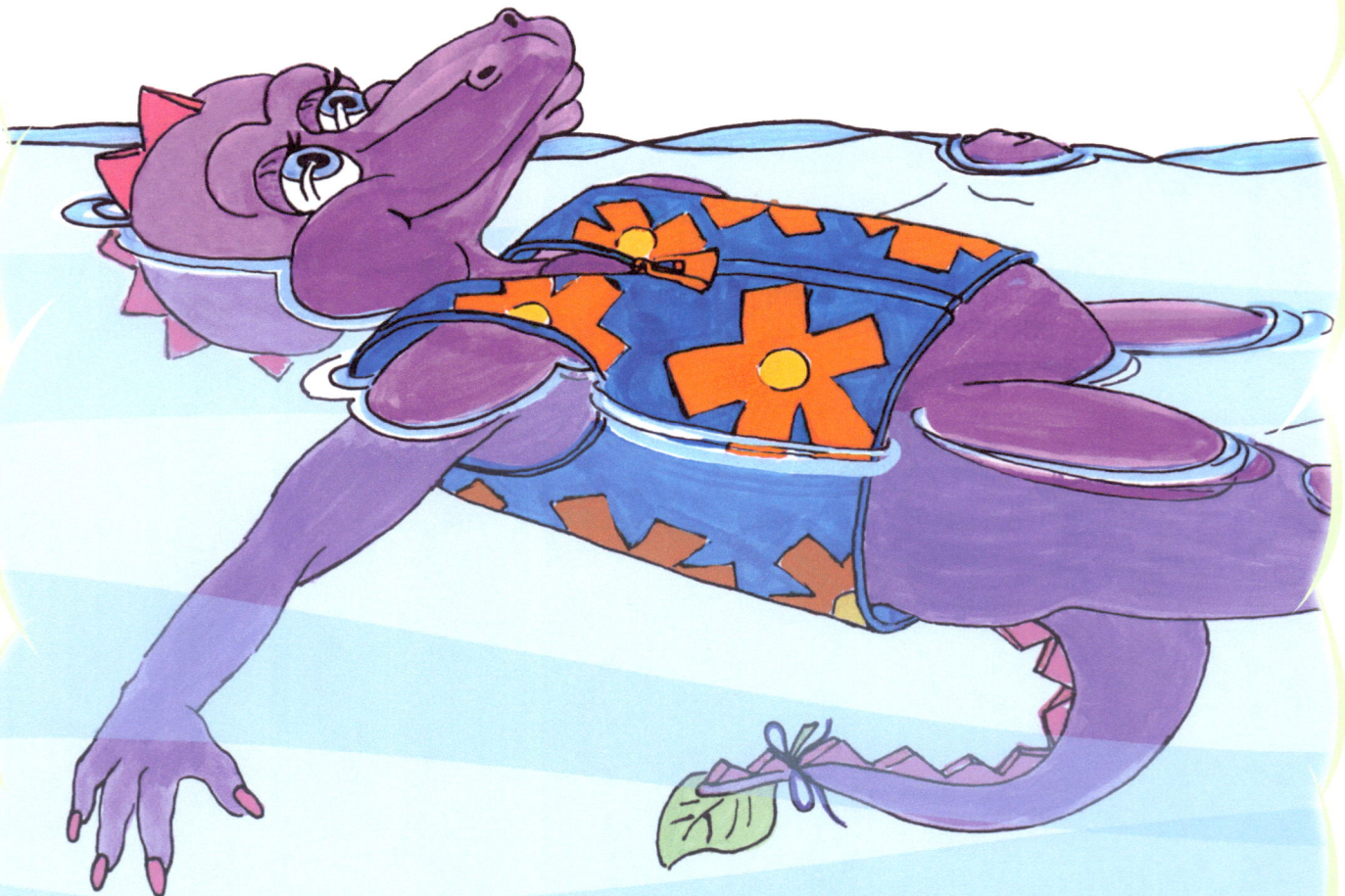

He taught them how to tread water with a life jacket on...

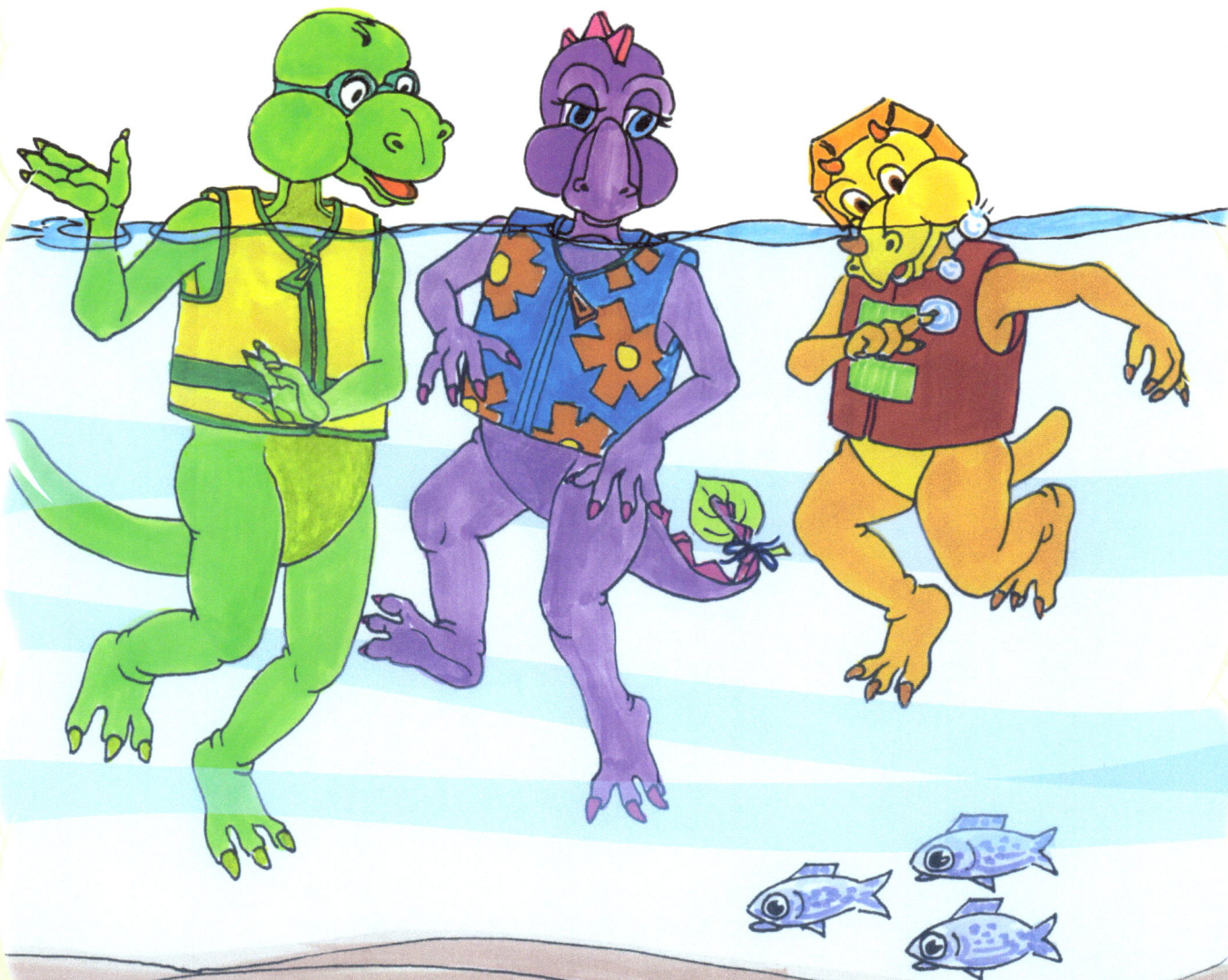

… and how to huddle to stay warm and safe in the water.

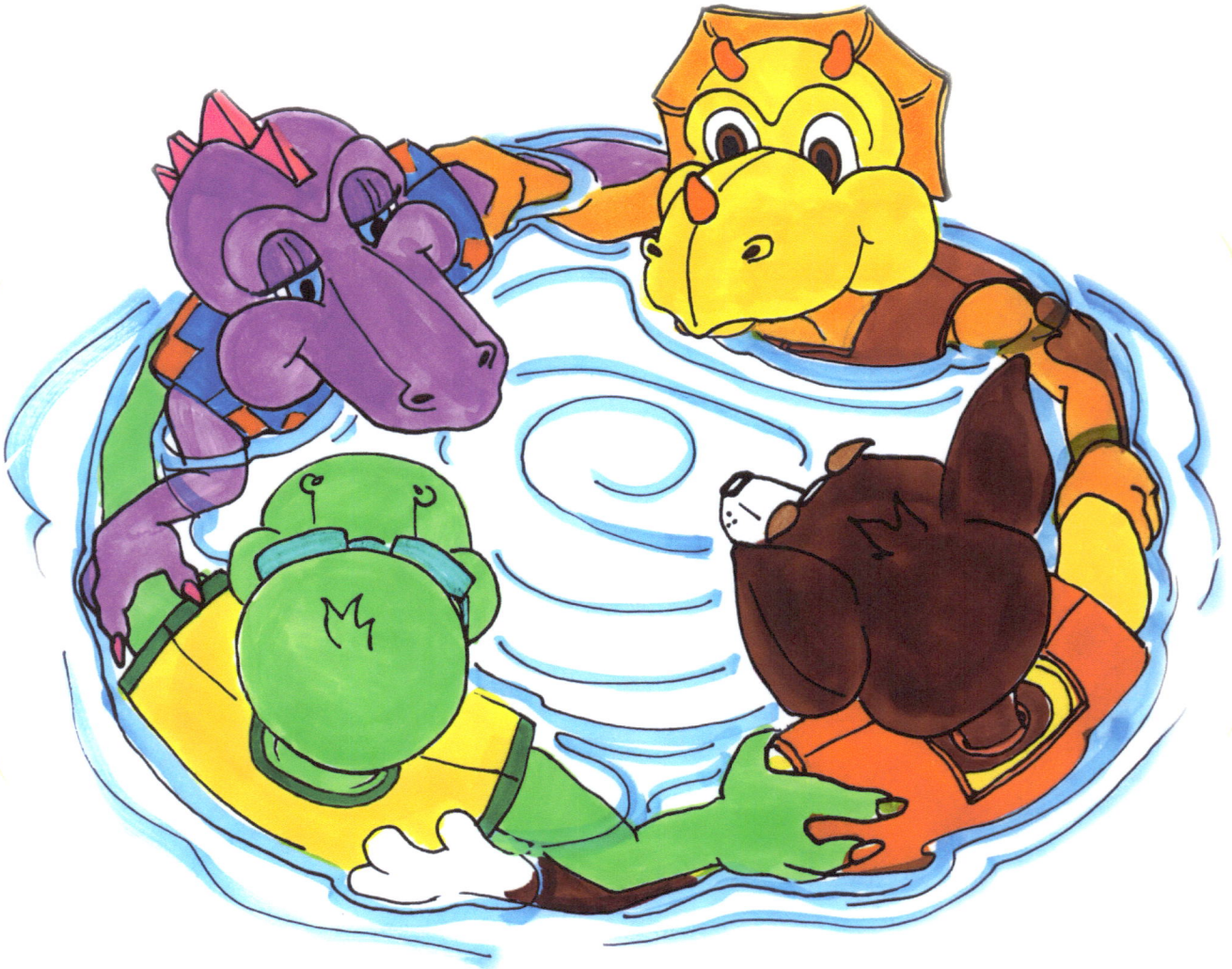

The whole lake was one big sea of huddling
dinosaurs. Everyone practiced and did very well.
Coco was a very good teacher, indeed!

Suddenly, there was a CRASH!
Mighty sounds came from
the canyon behind them!

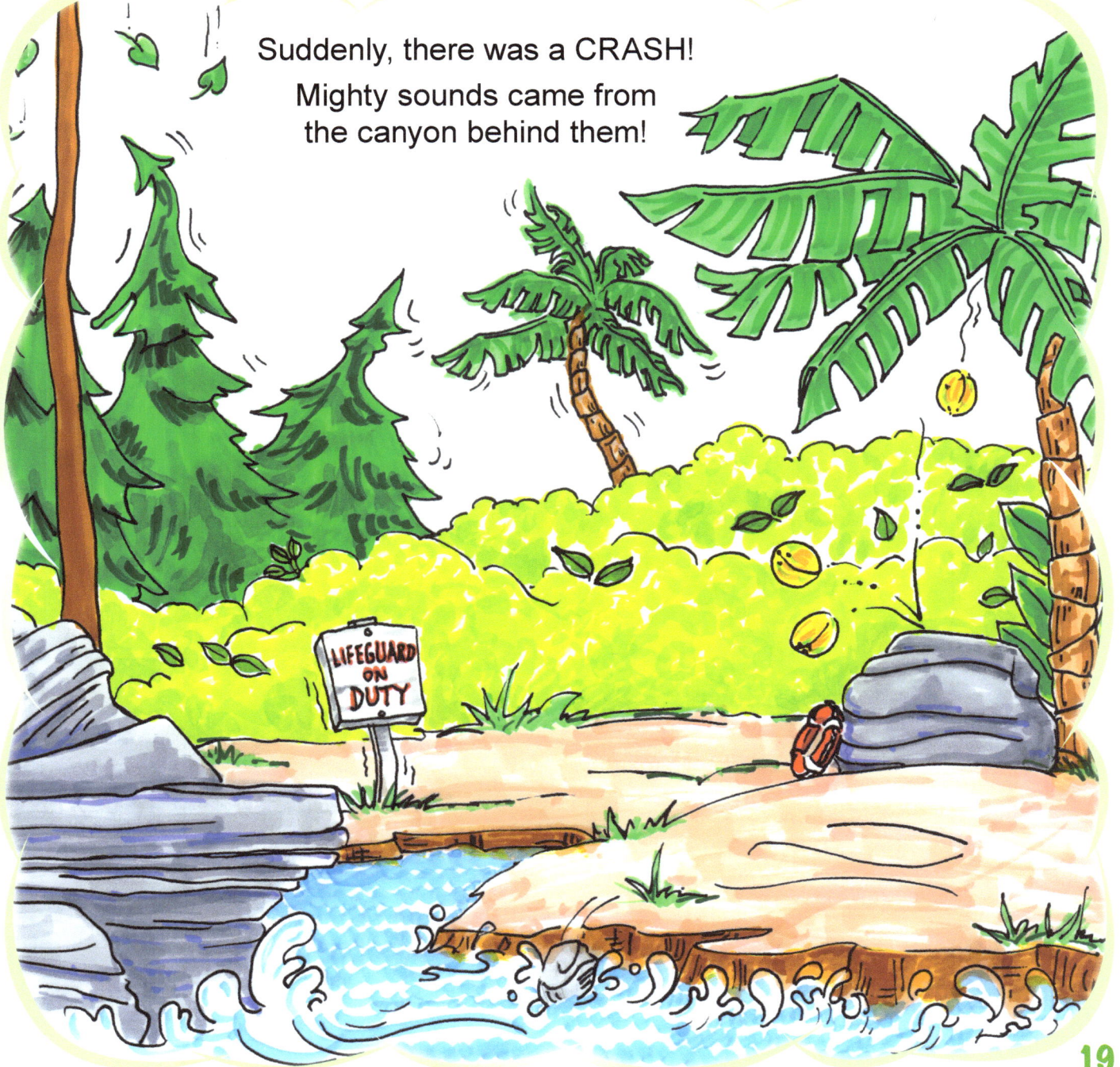

LIFEGUARD
ON
DUTY

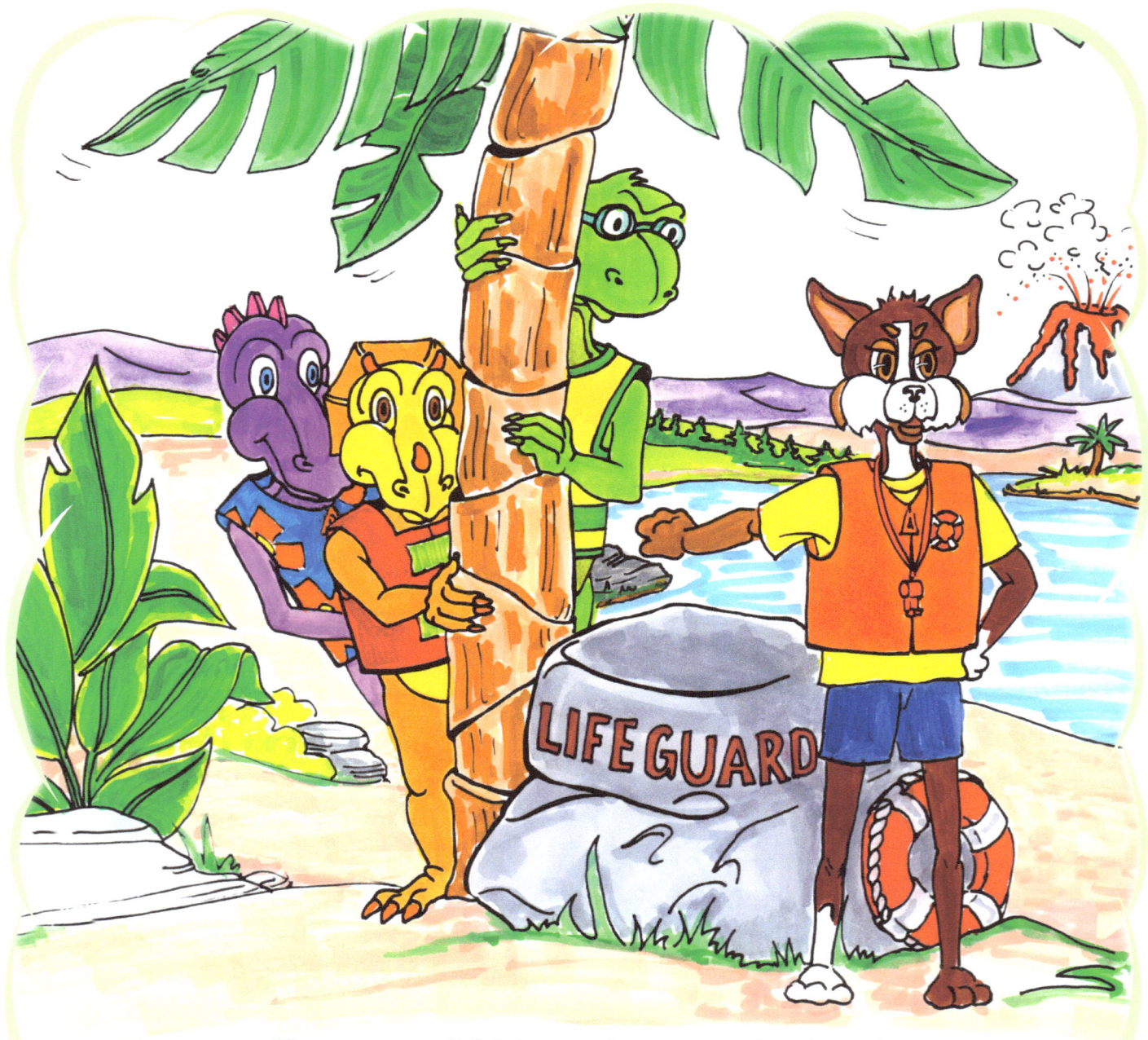

They were all frightened—except for Coco!

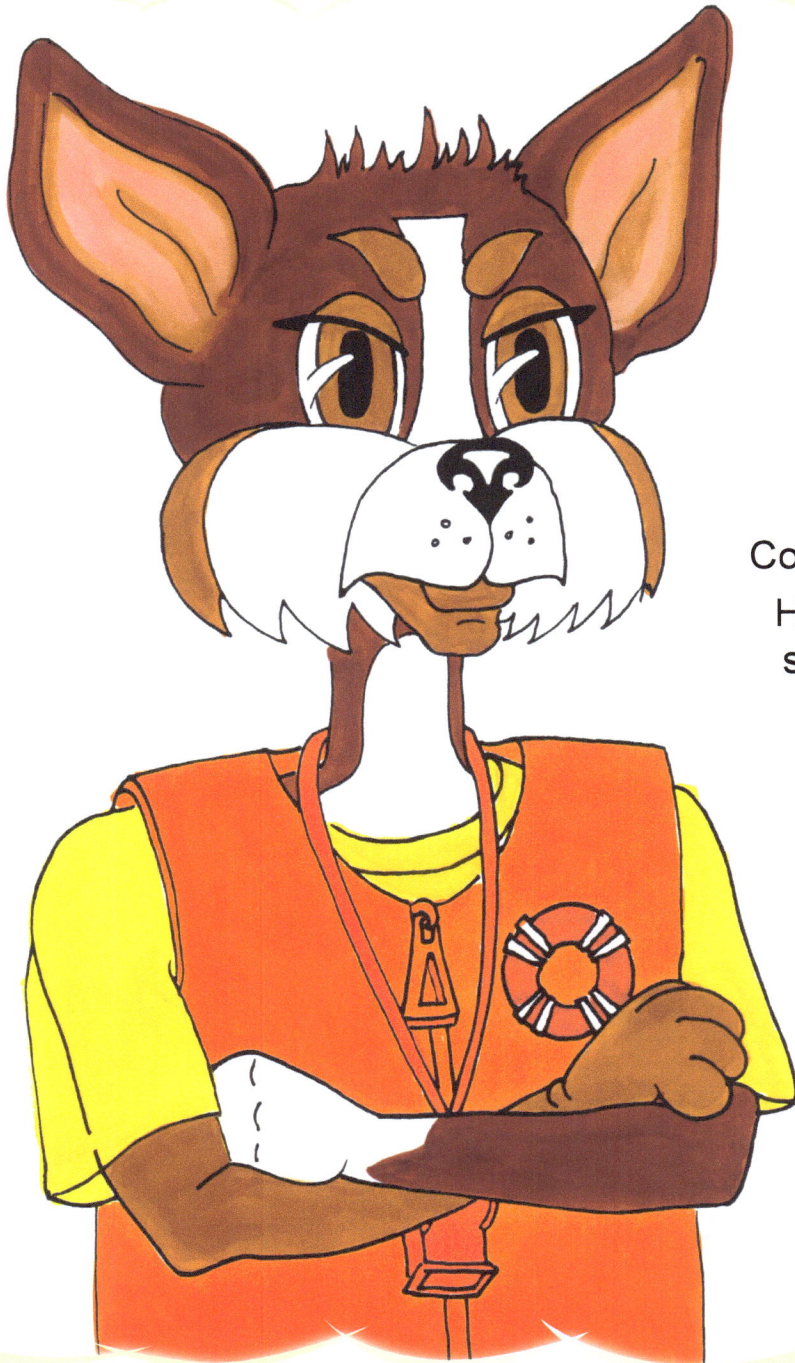

Coco stood his ground
He took this all very
seriously. He knew
he could keep
everyone safe.

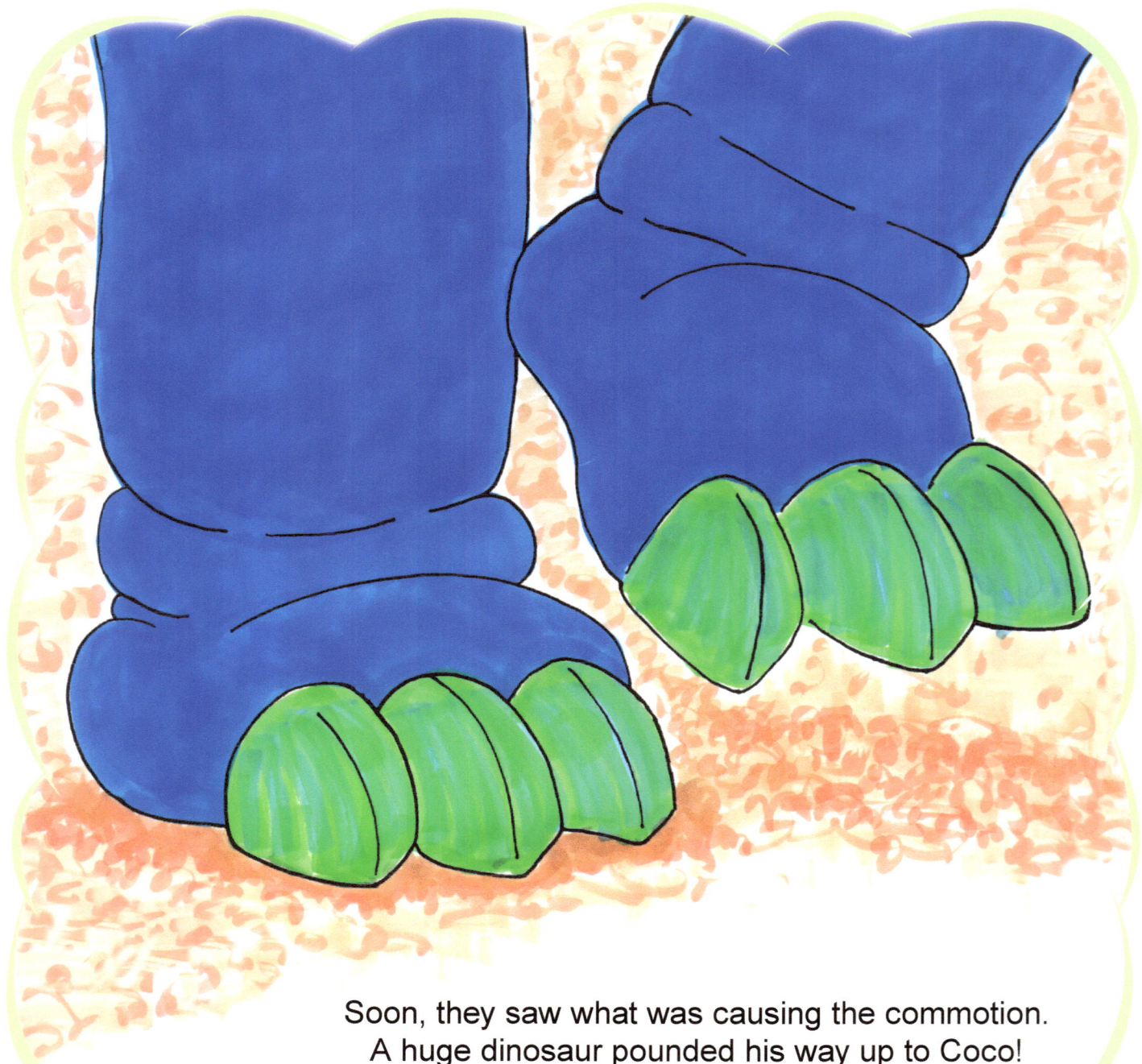

Soon, they saw what was causing the commotion.
A huge dinosaur pounded his way up to Coco!

The mighty dinosaur took a deep breath and said shyly, "My name is Otis. Would you teach me how to swim, too?"

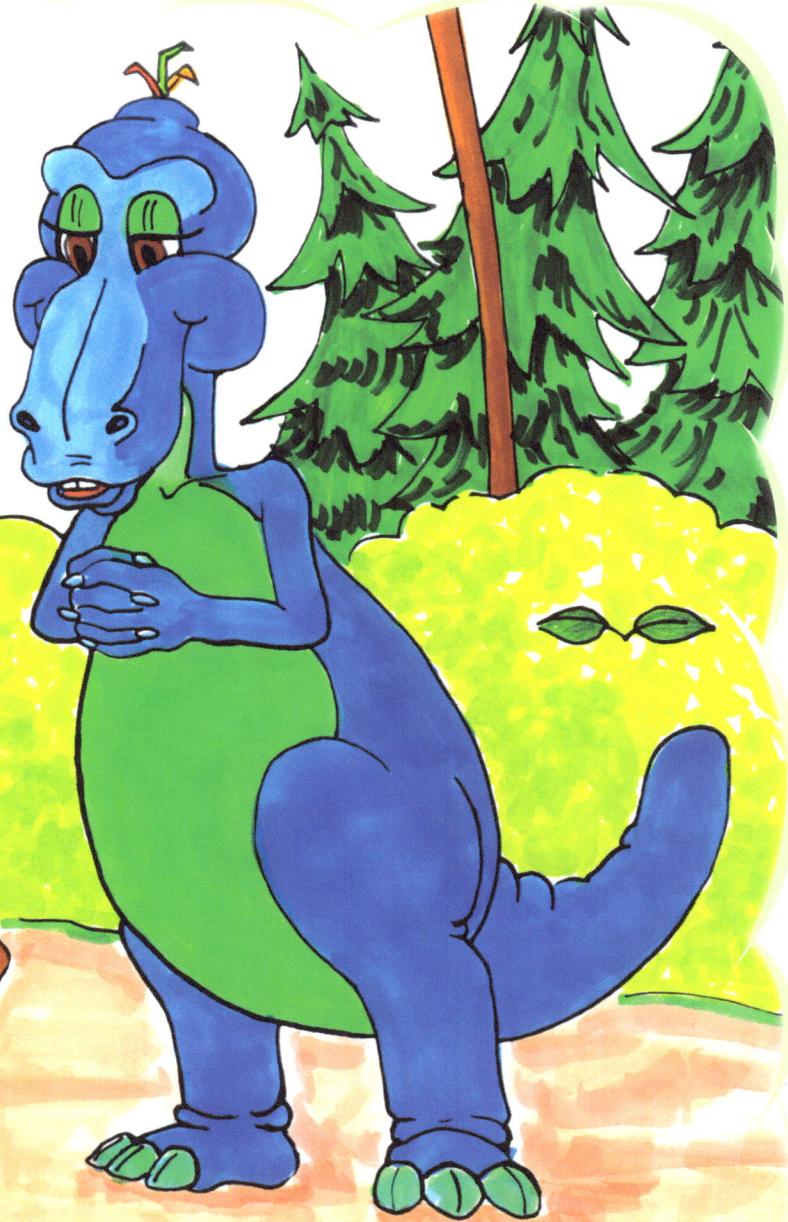

Everyone relaxed knowing they were not in danger.
Coco looked around at his students, then turned to Otis and said, "Of course!"

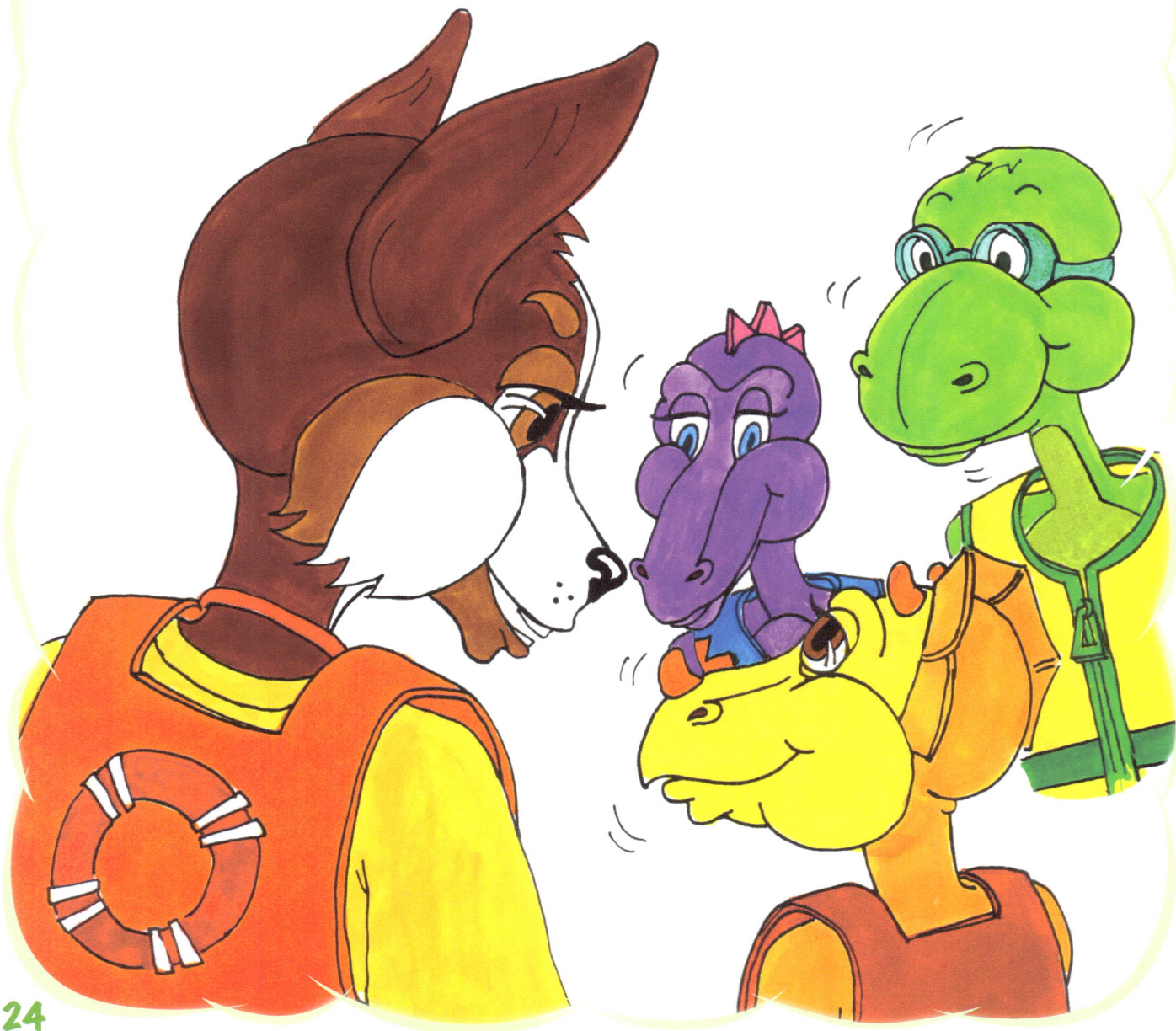

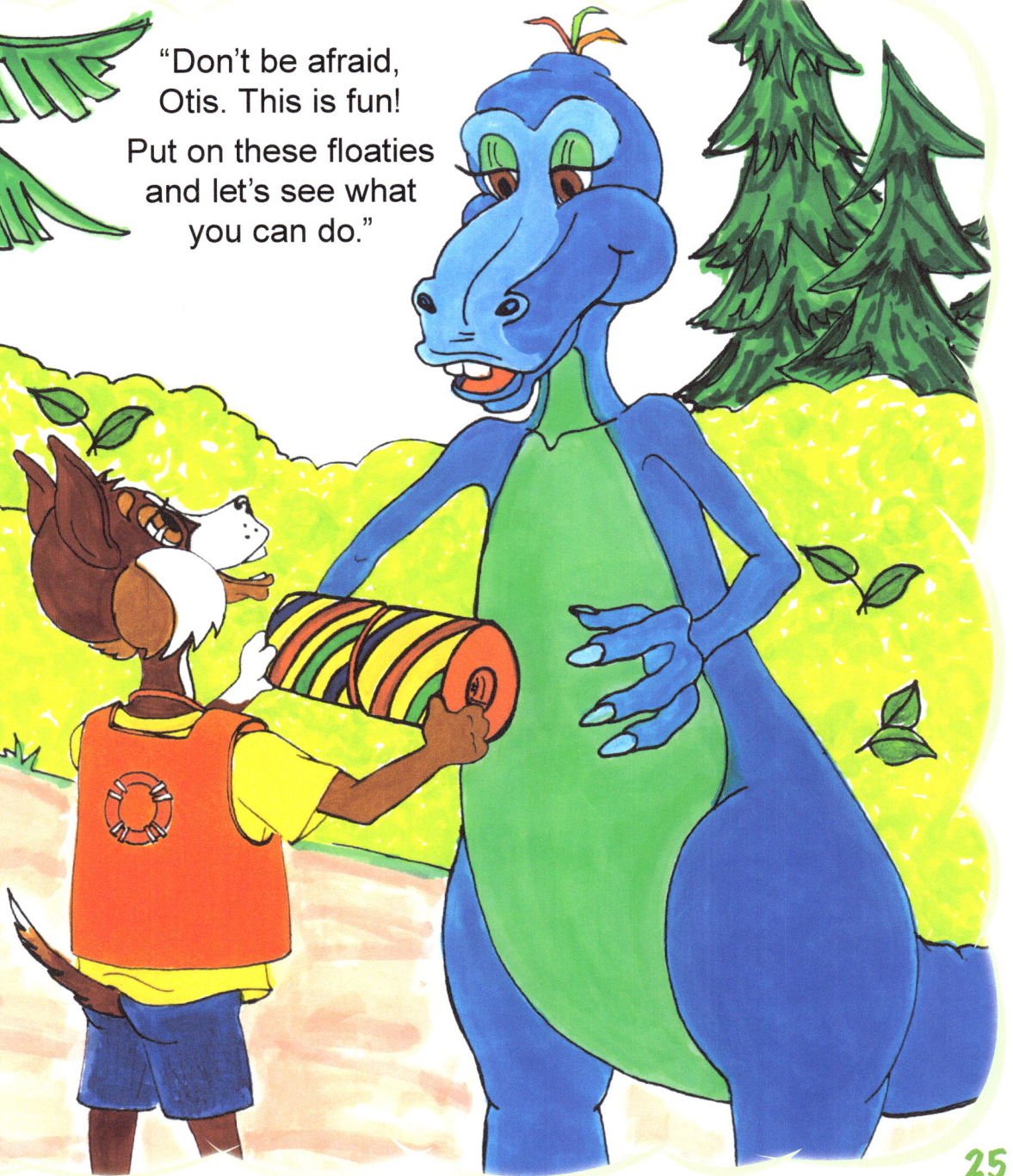

"Don't be afraid, Otis. This is fun!
Put on these floaties and let's see what you can do."

It was not long before all the youngsters
—including Otis—
were enjoying the water.

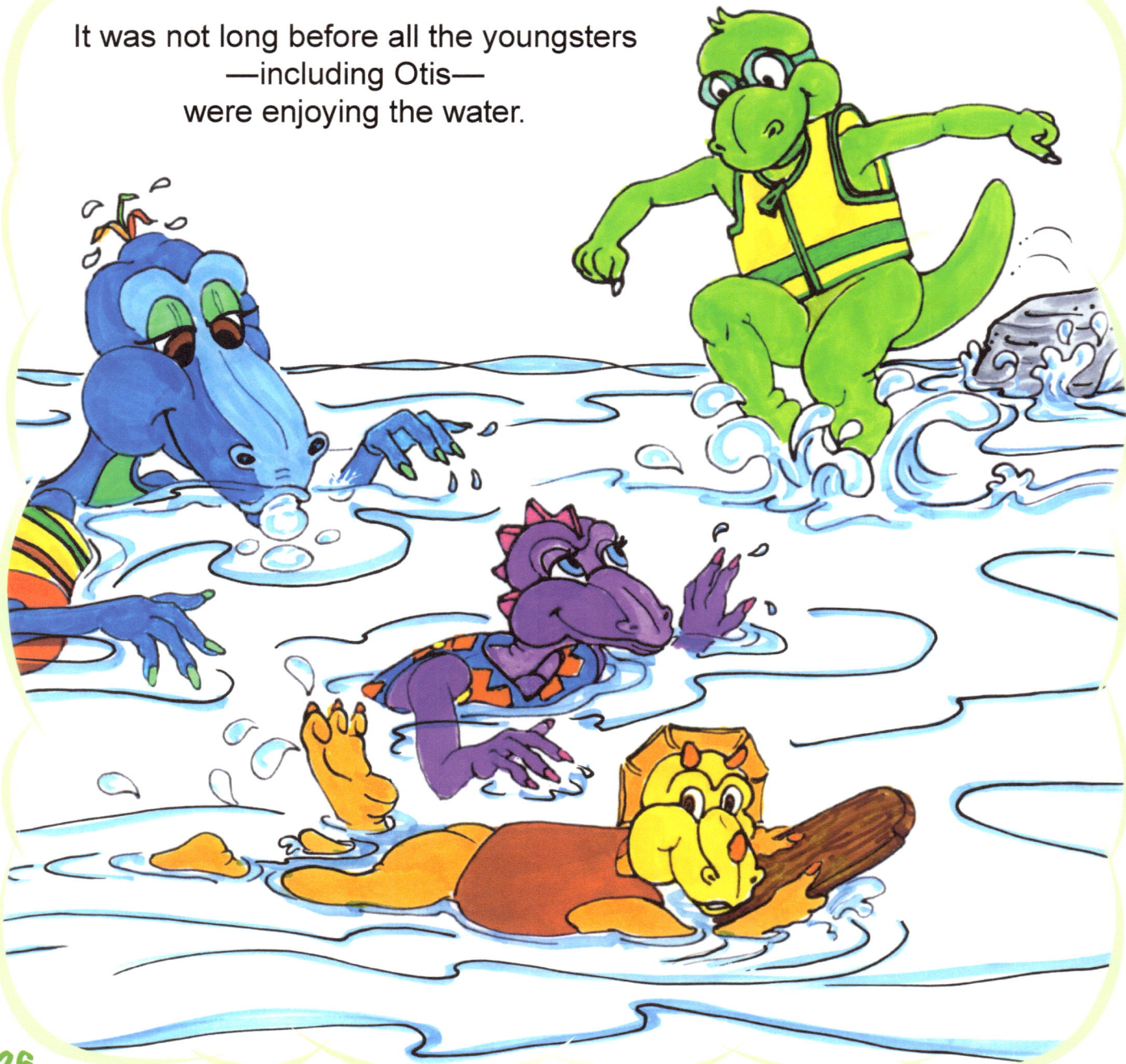

"May I come another day?" Otis asked.

All the young swimmers flapped their
tails on the water in agreement.
What a stir they made!

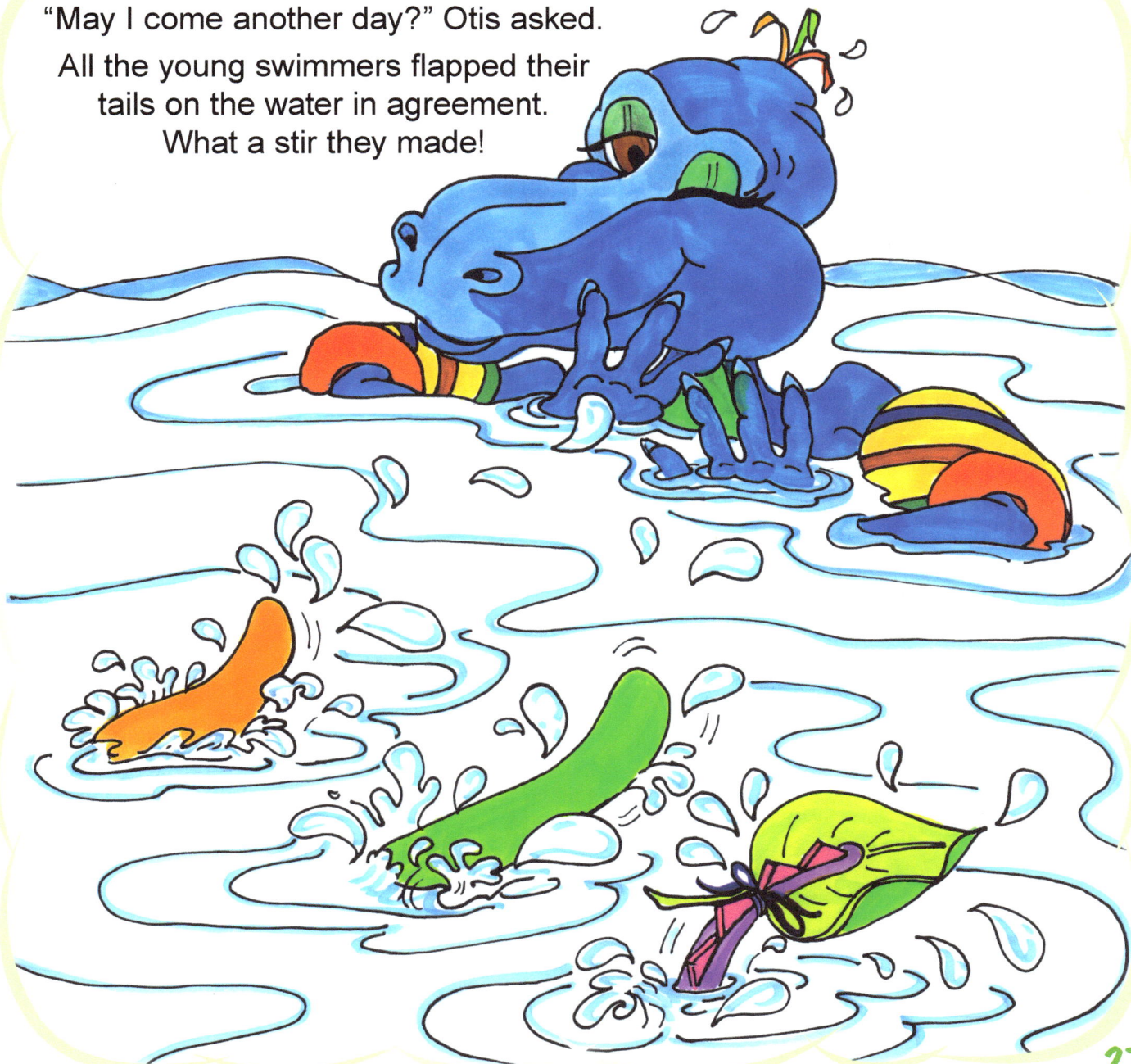

Coco blew his lifeguard whistle and called, "Everyone out of the water. It is time to go home!"

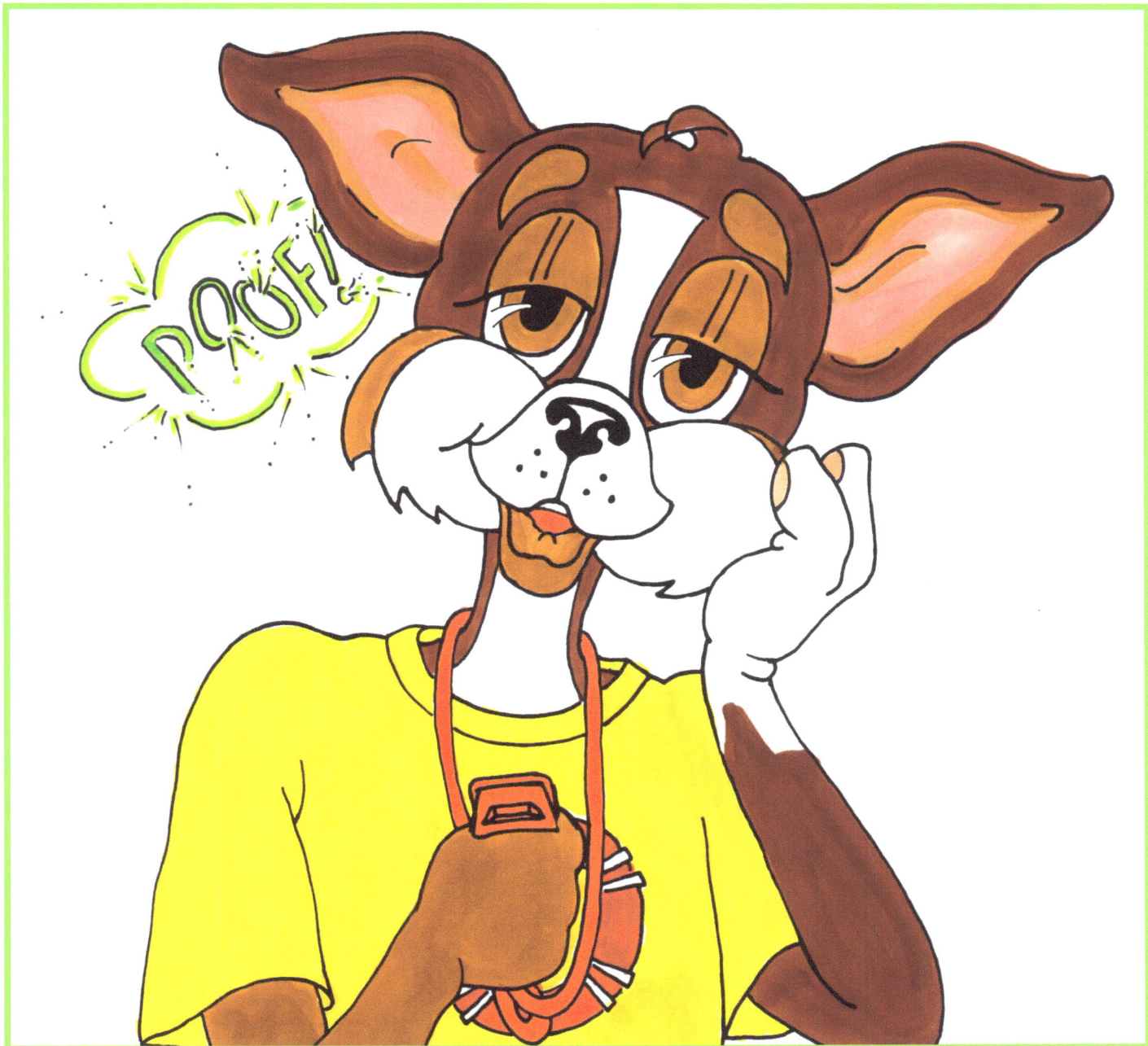

"Not just yet," Mrs. Jabbers said as Coco found himself standing on his desk.
His classmates giggled as he sat back down.

29

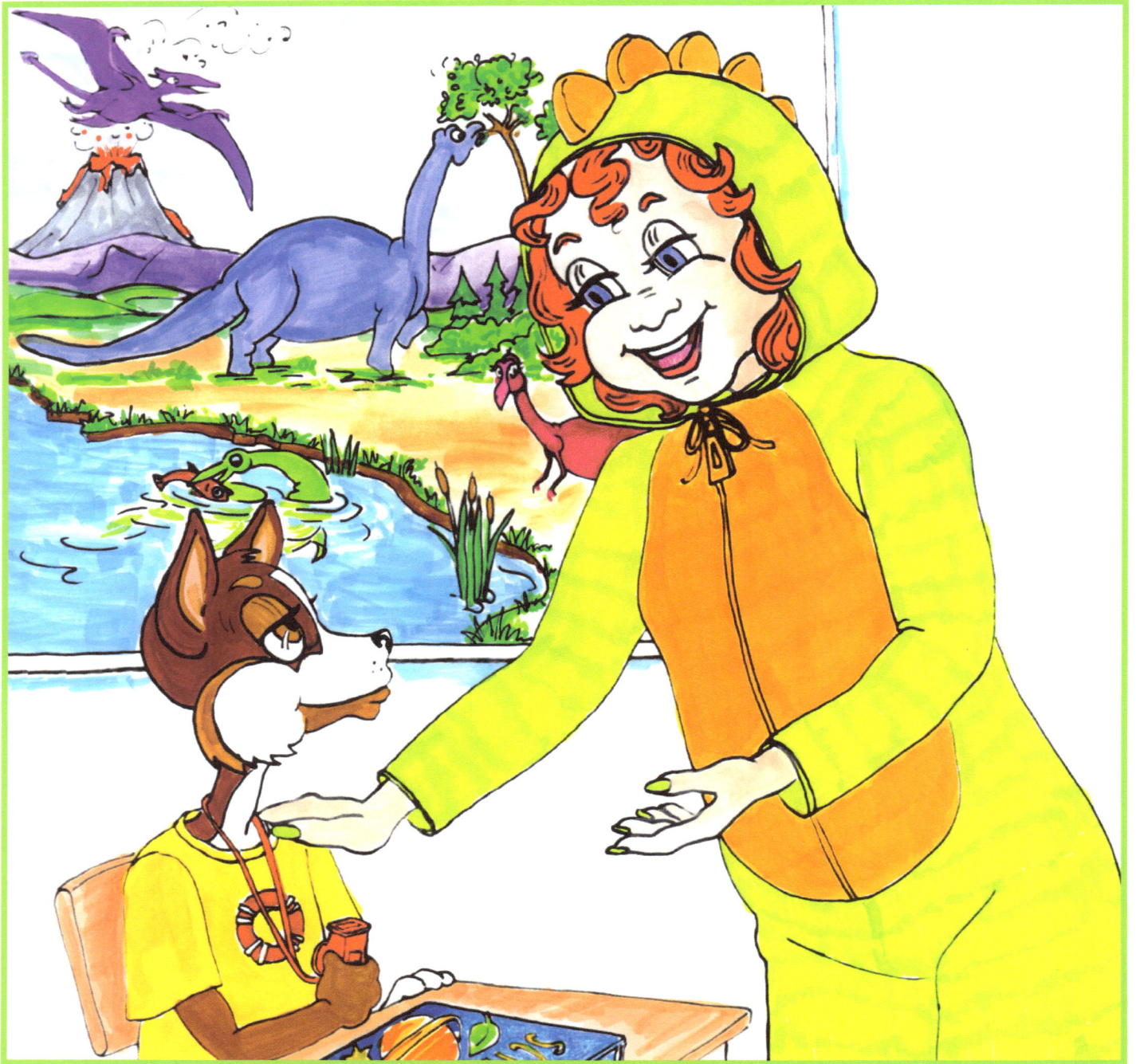

Mrs. Jabbers smiled and said, "Welcome back, Coco!"

A Special Message from Dr. B

While swimming and spending time outside is a lot of fun, it is very important to take good care of your health.

Here are some health tips to live by:

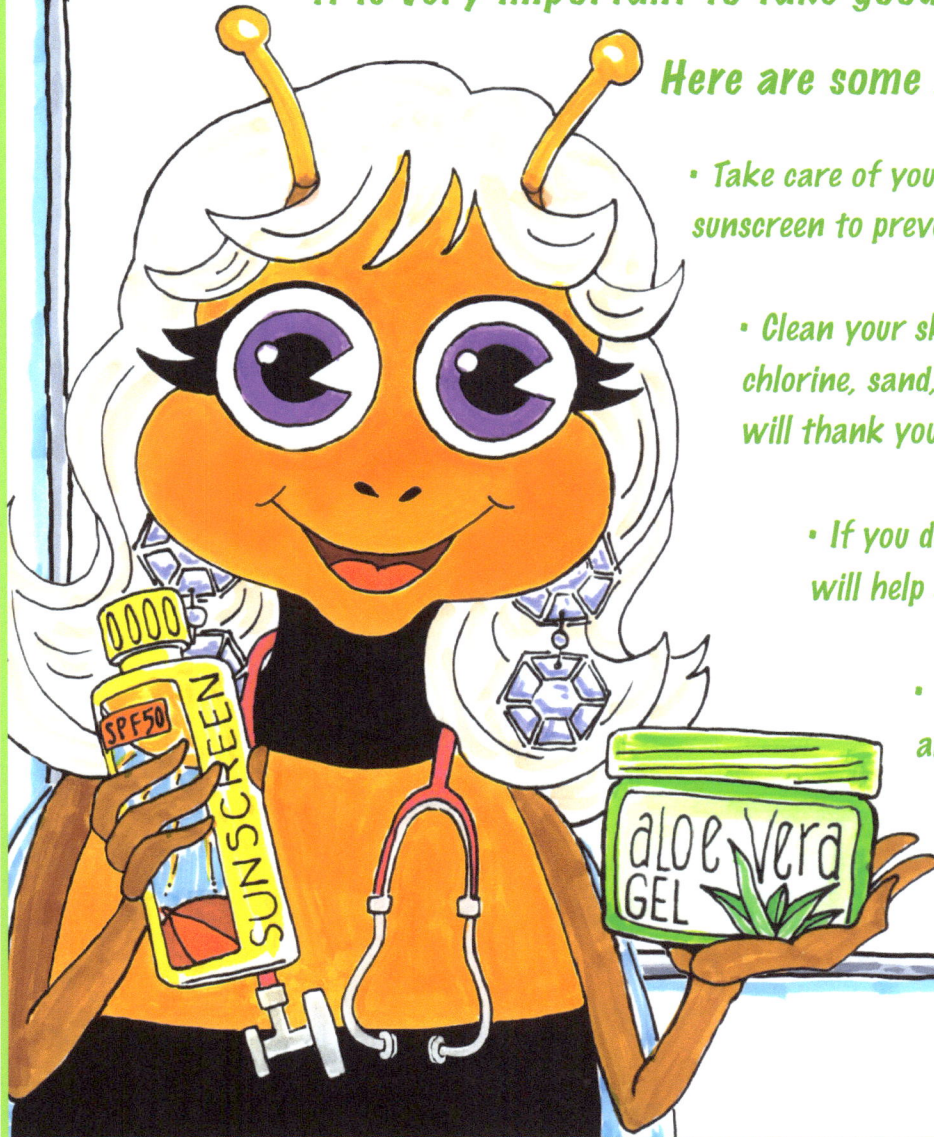

• Take care of your skin. Use good-quality sunscreen to prevent your skin from burning.

• Clean your skin to wash away sweat, dirt, chlorine, sand, and sunscreen. Your skin will thank you for it!

• If you do get a sunburn, aloe vera gel will help soothe the hurt.

• Protect your eyes. Wear hats and sunglasses.

• Spend time in the shade.

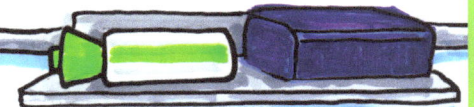

• Drink lots of water. Your cells need water to function properly.

• Eat lots of berries, colorful fruits, and vegetables. These foods have vitamins and minerals that your body needs to stay active and full of energy.

• Eat fruit instead of sugary snacks. Eating sugar can make you feel very tired. It robs your body of vitamins and minerals that you need to stay healthy and happy.

• Rest when you are tired. If you feel tired, it is good to take time to rest—especially if you are swimming or playing hard.

• Don't play too hard.

• Learn to control your breathing with meditation and breathing exercises.

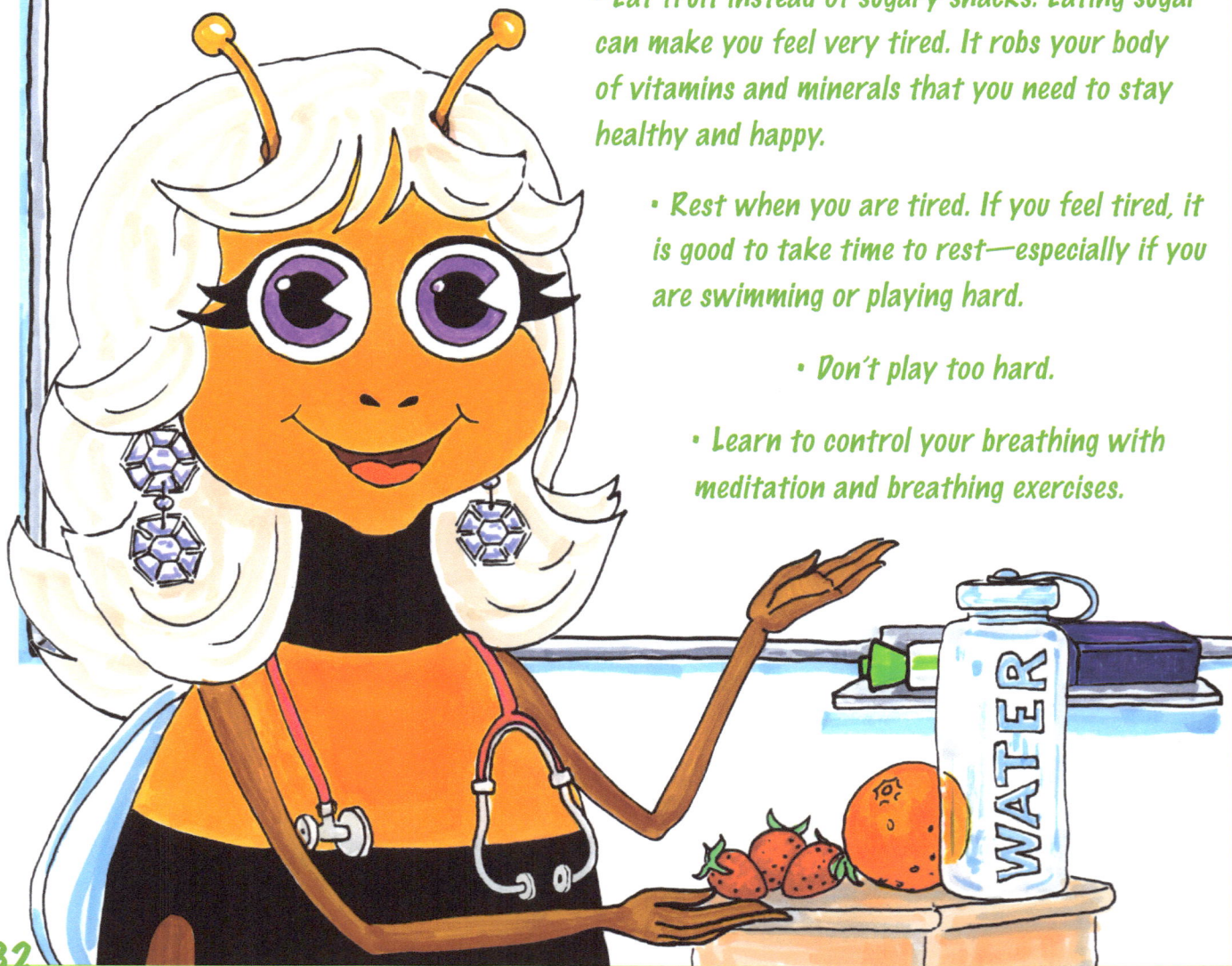

Do you want to know more about dinosaurs?
Here are some books you might enjoy:

• Norman, David. **The Illustrated Encyclopedia of Dinosaurs.** Crescent Books; New York. 1985.

• Norell, Mark. **Dinosaurs of the World.** Marshall Cavendish; Terrytown, New York. 1999.

• Parker, Steve. **The Age of Dinosaurs: The Carnosaurs.** Grolier Educational; Danbury, Connecticut. 2000.

• Zoehfeld, Kathleen Weidner. **Terrible Tyrannosaurus.** Harper Collin Publishers; New York, New York. 2001.

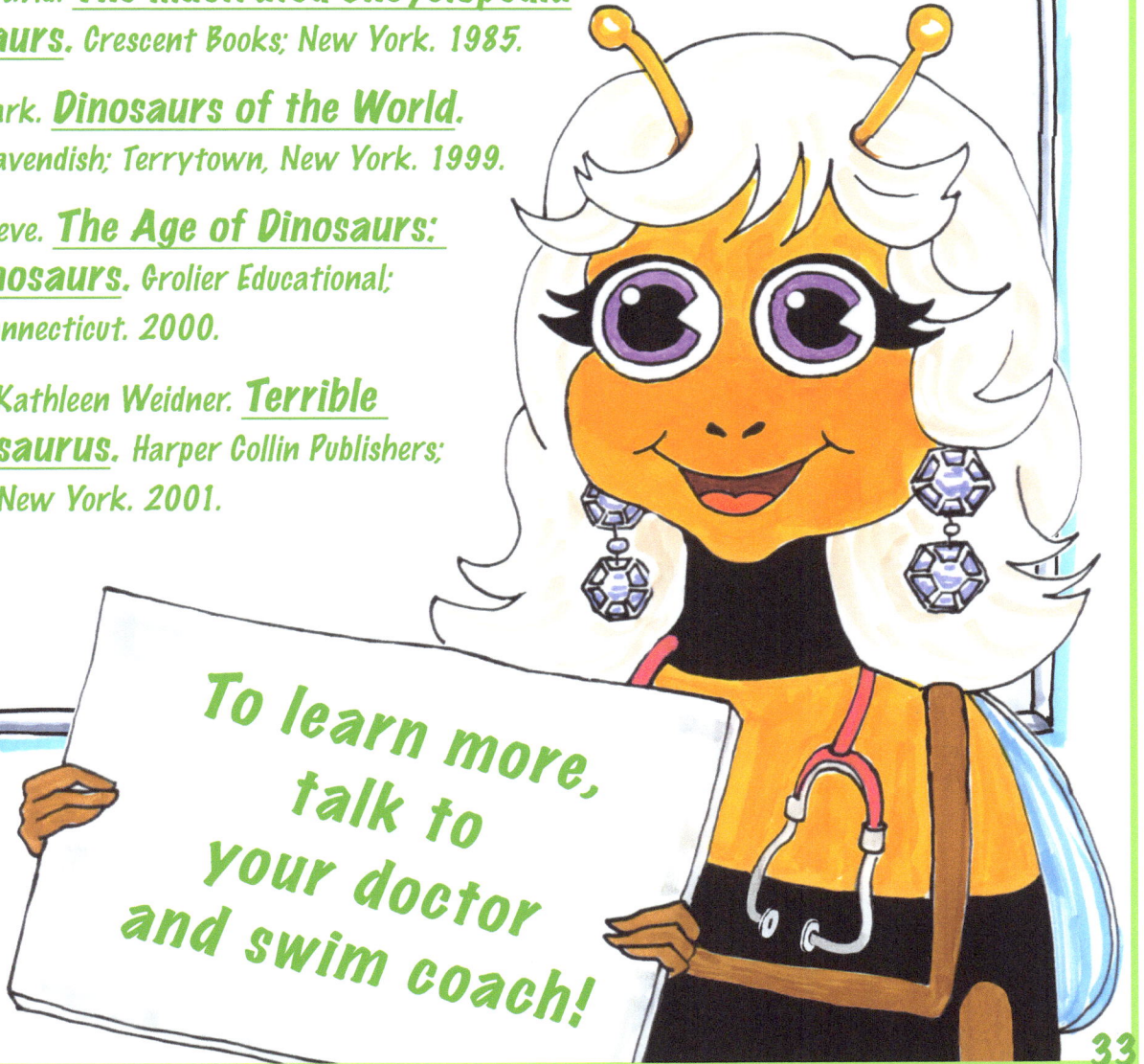

To learn more, talk to your doctor and swim coach!

www.ingramcontent.com/pod-product-compliance
Lightning Source LLC
Chambersburg PA
CBHW040933050426
42334CB00050B/93

9 780986 185069